UNDERSTANDING CLINICAL INVESTIGATIONS

For Baillière Tindall:

Senior Commissioning Editor: Ninette Premdas
Project Development Manager: Claire Wilson
Project Manager: Joannah Duncan and Andrew Palfreyman
Design: Judith Wright
Illustrations based on originals by Stephen White

SECOND EDITION

UNDERSTANDING CLINICAL INVESTIGATIONS

A QUICK REFERENCE MANUAL

Susan Skinner MAEducation DipNurseEd RCNT RGN

Senior Lecturer, Neonatal Health, Anglia Polytechnic University, Essex, UK

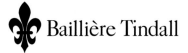

Baillière Tindall

EDINBURGH LONDON NEW YORK OXFORD PHILADELPHIA ST LOUIS SYDNEY TORONTO 2005

BAILLIÈRE TINDALL

An imprint of Elsevier Limited

First edition 1996
Reprinted 2000, 2002
Second edition 2005

ISBN 0 7020 2683 2

British Library Cataloguing in Publication Data
A catalogue record for this book is available from the British Library

Library of Congress Cataloging in Publication Data
A catalog record for this book is available from the Library of Congress

Notice
Knowledge and best practice in this field are constantly changing. As new research and experience broaden our knowledge, changes in practice, treatment and drug therapy may become necessary or appropriate. Readers are advised to check the most current information provided (i) on procedures featured or (ii) by the manufacturer of each product to be administered, to verify the recommended dose or formula, the method and duration of administration, and contraindications. It is the responsibility of the practitioner, relying on their own experience and knowledge of the patient, to make diagnoses, to determine dosages and the best treatment for each individual patient, and to take all appropriate safety precautions. To the fullest extent of the law, neither the publisher nor the author assumes any liability for any injury and/or damage.

The Publisher

ELSEVIER your source for books,
journals and multimedia
in the health sciences

www.elsevierhealth.com

The
Publisher's
policy is to use
**paper manufactured
from sustainable forests**

Printed in China

Contents

RB
37
565
2005

Acknowledgements

My thanks to Wendy Prescott and Rob Florer for their help and advice.

Introduction

Although many advances have been made since the first edition of this book appeared, the basic principles of monitoring and care have not changed. Clinical investigations are not theoretical exercises; they are often the precursor to life-changing events and the care that patients receive during this time must reflect this. In acknowledgement of nurses working to give this support to people in their care, I hope that this book supplies them with a constant source of easily accessed assistance.

Susan Skinner, 2005

Warning

All assessment values given in this book must be checked against your locally accepted normal values.

The measurements given in this book can only be accepted as normal values within the departments from which they were developed.

Please substitute locally accepted normal values into the text.

For the purposes of this book:
- 'Neonate' refers to an infant during the first week of life
- 'Child' refers to a person between infancy and the early teenage years
- 'Adult' refers to a person who is physically, fully mature.

The author acknowledges that these statements are broad, but the individualistic nature of clinical investigation and the specificity of results and measurements obtained, means that only generalisations can be used in a book of this type. Again, adapt the book to suit the profile of your own special types of patient.

ASSESSMENT OF PATIENTS

CARE OF PATIENTS

Most of us have experienced the fear and uncertainty when clinical investigations become necessary to check our own health or the health of friends and family. We have also experienced the feeling of relief, or dejection, when the test results are known. Remembering these feelings makes us better practitioners when patients rely on us for support during difficult times.

Prepare well and have all equipment ready before meeting the patient.

Give clear, simple explanations appropriate to the patient's level of understanding.

Worry causes thoughts to be diverted, so be prepared to repeat items more than once.

The patient must be made as comfortable as the procedure allows.

Work with an air of confidence; it helps you and it helps the patient.

Talk to the patient throughout, reporting on progress and giving assurance. If the nurse carrying out the procedure needs to concentrate and conversation is difficult, ask a colleague to assist.

Listen to the patient throughout. Try to make adjustments according to his or her request and reported discomforts.

An appraisal of the well-being of the patient should be made throughout.

Infection control measures should be properly enforced.

Factors that may alter the test result must be eliminated, or accounted for, during the initial preparations.

All specimen bottles must be properly and fully labelled.

Request forms must contain all relevant information.

MEETING THE SPECIAL NEEDS OF INFANTS AND CHILDREN

The newborn baby is vulnerable because of its size and immaturity. Methods to evaluate the risks of further compromising their health through investigative procedures must be in place.

Assessment methods are often restrictive, uncomfortable and even painful. They produce situations that would normally be avoided. Extra time and planning is needed to gain the child's trust and co-operation.

Parents should be fully informed on all aspects of the child's care.

If the parents are to be part of an assessment procedure, they should only be used as a support and comfort to the child. They should not become active participants restraining the child during any distressing aspects of the procedure.

CARE OF STAFF

Staff must protect themselves from harm, or from being exposed to risk from other sources. The risk factors associated with assessment methods must be recognised and full protective measures must be taken.

Pre-plan the procedure and follow the plan in practice.

Basic precautions for practice:
- Protective gloves should always be available and worn when there is a risk of contamination.
- Handwashing facilities must be available and used at the correct times prescribed by the procedure.
- Equipment and materials should be disposed of correctly and safely. Sharps must be properly disposed of after use.
- When radioactive materials and X-rays are part of the investigation procedure, staff must wear appropriate protective clothing. When a staff member is in regular contact with radioactive materials, a monitoring film badge should be worn at the waist.

The policies and procedures laid down by local authorised committees should be followed. This gives the practitioner recourse and protection when:
- The patient or practitioner is harmed by the technique.
- The procedure is brought into question by the patient or other staff.

- The Code of Professional Conduct appropriate to the practitioners' professional body, e.g. Nursing and Midwifery Council, must underpin all interventions.
- Staff must ensure that written consent is taken from the patient, or next of kin, before carrying out procedures that require this type of permission.
- Clear information and explanations should always be given to the patient. The patient will then know what to expect. The unexpected may give grounds for complaint.
- Staff should listen to the patient's remarks and complaints. It will help to avoid future repercussions.

INTERFERING FACTORS FOR CLINICAL INVESTIGATIONS

Abnormal results identified during clinical assessment may reflect factors that are associated with the patient's life rather than being a cause for concern. There are many influences acting on the body to produce deviations from expected norms, for example:

- Food – the nutritional status of a patient is a strong influence on many tests. Dieting will produce a urine that will test positive for ketones, yet the presence of ketones in other circumstances would be a serious consideration when evaluating a patient's health. Blood glucose variations are synchronous with meal times.

- Age – ageing has a detrimental effect on all systems and tissues of the body. These will need to be considered when a clinical picture is assessed. Sex hormone values will need to be evaluated according to the age of the patient.

- Drugs – drugs are designed to interfere with or change physiological processes. It is therefore inevitable that they will have an impact on some clinical investigations. Pharmacology books have numerous lists of changes in assessment values that can be associated with specific drugs. An example of this is the decreased measured prothrombin time associated with prescribed oral contraceptives.

- Time of day – the importance of the biorhythms on hormone and other tissue secretions is a matter of current research. Growth hormone is an example of this. It is secreted in regular bursts at preset times throughout the day with the largest burst of the hormone being secreted during the early part of sleep at night. As expected, the amount of growth hormone secreted and considered as a normal value will additionally be affected by the age of the patient.

- Body mass – the measurement of body mass and the estimation of normal standard values will always have to be set within the considerations of age and gender. Other influences affecting the measurements taken can include drug therapies, disturbances in metabolic rate, poor health and the appetite for food. Examples of these differences are the effects of long-term steroid therapy when assessing a patient with inflammatory disease or young athletes who take unprescribed anabolic steroids.

- Geographical area – adaptation of patients to their local environment may affect the normal values expected to be returned, when clinical investigations are carried out.

- The conditions under which the specimen was taken, or the use of poor collection techniques, may cause the results to be unreliable. For this reason results must be considered within the context of previously measured personal values or against previously measured baseline values.

TEMPERATURE

NORMAL MEASUREMENT

The core temperature of the body should measure 37°C.

PROCEDURE

A variety of thermometers are available:
- Electronic thermometers
- Disposable heat-sensitive strips.

The technique and site used to measure body temperature will depend on the patient and the design of the thermometer.

Core temperature is usually measured at body sites where blood vessels are near to the surface of the skin or mucous membranes:
- Under the tongue
- Inside the rectum
- Between the skin folds of the axilla.

Some types of thermometer specify other body areas to be used for measurement.
- This nursing procedure must follow local policy guidelines.
- The body area used and the type of thermometer chosen should depend completely on the safety and comfort of the patient.
- The same site should be used each time the patient has a temperature taken.
- The axilla should be dry before the thermometer is placed between the skin fold as dampness will affect the recording.
- Each technique used to take temperature carries its own hygienic considerations for the nurse to respond to.
- A knowledge of the anatomy of the rectum must precede the taking of a rectal temperature.
- Routine rectal temperature recordings on babies and children are no longer acceptable. If circumstances demand that the rectum is to be used, parental consent to the procedure should be obtained.

PURPOSE

To measure the core body temperature and use this information to assess the presence and progress of disease.

A measured temperature outside of the given normal range will be an indication of disease or environmental stress from heat or cold.

Cell metabolism operates at maximum efficiency when the body temperature is within normal limits and adjustment mechanisms exist to maintain the temperature at its correct value. Temperature constantly alters within a normal range. In normal circumstances it will fall to its lowest in the morning and rise to its highest point in the evening.

As leucocytes, or white blood cells, become damaged in their work against invading organisms they release pyrogens. Pyrogens reset the body temperature control in the hypothalamus to a higher core temperature, stimulating a reaction to conserve or manufacture body heat to meet the new set temperature point. A rise in body temperature is initiated and signs of feverishness will be seen.

A body temperature above 41°C (hyperthermia) will damage brain cells and blood vessels. A measured temperature below 35°C is described as hypothermia. A temperature lower than 32°C will become fatal if not treated.

NORMAL PHYSIOLOGY

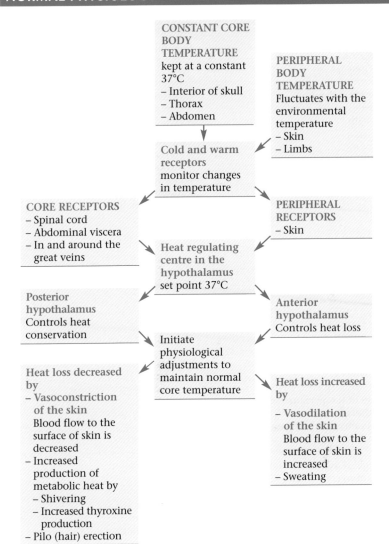

CONSTANT CORE BODY TEMPERATURE kept at a constant 37°C
– Interior of skull
– Thorax
– Abdomen

PERIPHERAL BODY TEMPERATURE Fluctuates with the environmental temperature
– Skin
– Limbs

Cold and warm receptors monitor changes in temperature

CORE RECEPTORS
– Spinal cord
– Abdominal viscera
– In and around the great veins

PERIPHERAL RECEPTORS
– Skin

Heat regulating centre in the hypothalamus set point 37°C

Posterior hypothalamus Controls heat conservation

Anterior hypothalamus Controls heat loss

Heat loss decreased by
– Vasoconstriction of the skin
  Blood flow to the surface of skin is decreased
– Increased production of metabolic heat by
  – Shivering
  – Increased thyroxine production
– Pilo (hair) erection

Initiate physiological adjustments to maintain normal core temperature

Heat loss increased by

– Vasodilation of the skin
  Blood flow to the surface of skin is increased
– Sweating

REASONS FOR ABNORMAL VALUES

RAISED TEMPERATURE	LOWERED TEMPERATURE
Pyrexia	**Hypothermia**
Hyperpyrexia	
Hot environment – Climate – Hot bath	Cold environment – Climate – Water
	Cold weather in conjunction with – Poor nutrition – Alcohol – Elderly – Immobility – Hypothyroidism
Unable to lose heat through evaporation from skin – Hot humid climate	
Raised body metabolism – Exercise	
Tissue trauma – Thrombosis – Auto-immune disease – Infarction – Malignancy	
Raising of temperature set point in hypothalamus – Viral or bacterial infection – Allergy	
Damage to hypothalamus – Neurosurgery – Cerebral oedema – Tumour	
Suppression of hypothalamus – Anaesthesia	Artificial cooling prior to surgery
Prior to ovulation	Immediately following birth, the temperature of the baby will drop. The temperature will stabilise within 7–10 hours.

ASSOCIATED INVESTIGATIONS

Related pages

Pulse rate and volume	Cell metabolism produces heat. The pulse rate will rise as the metabolic rate of cells increases. The pulse rate will slow when hypothermia decreases the metabolic rate.	10
Respirations	An increased metabolic rate will need an increased supply of oxygen to fuel the additional energy demands of the cells. Respirations will become more rapid. A low temperature and a decrease in metabolic rate will reduce the amount of oxygen needed by the cells. Respirations will become slower and shallower.	129
Blood pH measurement	The metabolic and respiratory changes described above will alter the acid/base balance of the body.	150
Differential white cell count	To determine the type of agent that is causing the hypothalamic temperature set point to rise.	44
Urine volume and specific gravity	To detect dehydration either from excessive sweating, or inadequate fluid intake.	173 180
Neurological observations	The extremes of hyperpyrexia and hypothermia can each cause neurological disturbances.	245
Electrocardiographic monitoring	The extremes of hyperpyrexia and hypothermia will each cause cardiac arrhythmias.	24
Blood sodium levels	Sodium will be lost during profuse, prolonged sweating.	97
Thyroid function tests	Hypothyroidism will decrease the metabolic rate and the ability of the body to generate heat. Hyperthyroidism will increase the metabolic rate and the amount of body heat produced.	91

CONSIDERATIONS FOR CARE

RAISED TEMPERATURES

A feverish patient will be suffering the uncomfortable process of generating heat by shivering and conserving heat by vasoconstriction, to reach and maintain the higher hypothalamic temperature set point. When the new temperature has been reached and exceeded, the body will lose heat by sweating and vasodilation, in its attempt to stabilise an abnormal temperature.

This alternating process of heating and cooling will mean that the nurse must be sensitive to the patient's requirements, by regulating the environmental temperature around the patient:

- Removal of bedclothes and clothing is soothing when the patient is trying to lose heat, but it will be stressful when he or she is shivering to produce more heat. A light cover should be available when necessary, to be removed when no longer needed.
- If a fan is used to circulate cool air, it must be placed at a distance from and directed away from the patient, and the other patients in the ward.
- The pillow should be turned frequently to give a cool place to lie the head. Fresh bed linen should be available, especially if the patient is sweating excessively.
- Skin hygiene will be important.

Cool drinks should be given if permitted:

- To prevent dehydration, especially when there is profuse sweating.
- To refresh the patient.

An intravenous infusion may be necessary when an inadequate amount of fluid is taken by mouth. Sodium supplement may also be necessary.

The raised metabolic rate will become exhausting. Rest is therefore essential.

The regular recording of the temperature may gradually show a cyclical pattern of raised and lowered body temperature. This may help with the diagnosis of the underlying condition.

Prescribed drugs may include:

- Antipyretics to reduce the temperature. These are especially important to children under 5 years of age as the high temperature may cause a febrile convulsion.
- Analgesics: the antipyretic may have analgesic properties.
- Antibiotics, if an infection is the cause of the raised temperature.

LOWERED TEMPERATURES

Hypothermic patients will need slow, careful warming:

- They should be nursed in a warm environment.
- A covering that will insulate and conserve body heat.
- Drinks should be warmed, as should intravenous fluids, if they are prescribed.

The skin will be in a prolonged state of vasoconstriction, diminishing its oxygen supply. This will weaken the tissues. The skin should not be rubbed and frequent pressure area care will be needed to avoid injury. The skin should be examined for areas of frostbite.

Cardiac monitoring will detect cardiac arrhythmias precipitated by the hypothermia.

The patient may be confused or unconscious. Neurological observations may then be of value.

When hypothermia is caused by poor social conditions, help and advice should be given to the patient prior to discharge.

PULSE

REFERENCE RANGE

Adult: 60–80 beats/min

Child: 70–120 beats/min. This can only be taken as a general value.

A child's pulse gradually slows with increasing age. Each child should therefore be assessed according to age and development.

Neonate: 120–160 beats/min

PROCEDURE

The procedure should be carried out according to local policy.

It is important that the patient is comfortable and relaxed.

It may be better to take the pulse of young children as they sleep. For this reason the site chosen for taking the pulse must depend on the patient's condition and the reason for recording the pulse rate.

PURPOSE

To ensure that the heart is beating at an appropriate rate.

The pulse should also be examined for abnormalities of rhythm and volume.

The pulse gives an indirect measurement of heart rate. It also provides information about the health of the heart and circulatory system.

It is the heart that provides the driving force that perpetuates the continuous circuit of blood around the body. As the heart beats, an intermittent pulse pressure is relayed in waves through the arterial system. The contraction of the cardiac ventricles initiates this wave of pressure that expands and retracts the walls of the arteries. These waves are felt at various points on the body as pulses.

When a pulse is taken, it is the waves of pressure passing along the arterial walls that is assessed, not the movement of blood through the arteries.

Regular recording of the pulse can provide a pattern from which to draw information about a patient's state of health. Few conclusions can be drawn from a single recording.

APICAL BEAT

NORMAL MEASUREMENT

The heart beat and the peripheral pulses should be identical in rate and volume.

PROCEDURE

The procedure to compare the heart rate with the radial or other peripheral pulses should be carried out according to local policy and procedure.

Two nurses must carry out the procedure.

One nurse counts the apex beat of the heart using a stethoscope; the other nurse simultaneously counts the peripheral pulse, usually the radial pulse.

The same watch or clock should be used by both nurses.

The start and finish time must be agreed before the counting begins.

PURPOSE

To ensure that the heart rate is identical to the peripheral pulse rate.

The heart beat originates in the sino-atrial node, a group of cells sited in the right atrium of the heart. The sino-atrial node produces nerve impulses that travel through the muscular walls of the atria, and cause them to contract.

As the atria contract, the nerve impulses continue to travel down through the septum of the heart.

The impulses pass through the walls of the ventricles causing them to contract in turn. This creates the apex beat heard in the midclavicular line at the fifth intercostal space. This position may be altered by disease.

The difference in pressure created by the ventricles contracting and the ventricles at rest creates a pulse of pressure that travels through the aorta and arterial system to be felt at the peripheral pulses.

Heart disease or vascular disease can block the waves of pulse pressure from travelling through the arterial system. The pressure wave will not reach the peripheral pulse. This will give a discrepancy between the heart rate count and the pulse rate count.

Conditions creating reduced peripheral pulses include:
- Co-arctation of the aorta
- Occlusive disease of the aorta.

Infants under one year old. The small peripheral blood vessels make counting the radial pulse difficult. For accuracy, the heart rate should be counted at the apex of the heart, using a stethoscope. For this procedure to be successful, the baby should be quiet and still, asleep if possible.

Femoral pulses of the newborn are examined for their presence and synchronicity. Absent femoral pulses indicates congenital co-arctation of the aorta.

NORMAL PHYSIOLOGY

Blood flows through the heart.

▼

Left ventricle contracts expelling blood into the aorta.
The rate of contraction is determined by the cardiac centre in the medulla of the brain.

▼

A pulse of pressure is generated by the contracting ventricles.

▼

The pulse pressure is the **difference in pressure** exerted on arterial blood between
– The ventricles contracting – **systole** (120 mmHg)
– The ventricles at rest – **diastole** (80 mmHg).

▼

The pulse of pressure moves from the heart into the walls of the aorta.

▼

The aorta expands as the pressure in the aortic wall rises.

▼

The aortic valve shuts, to keep the expelled blood in the aorta, from where it starts its systemic circulation.

▼

The pressure in the wall of the proximal aorta begins its movement as a wave travelling down the muscular aortic wall.

▼

This wave of pulse pressure continues to track its path through the arterial vessel walls until it fades in the arterial capillary system.

Normal physiology

Points of the body where the pulse can be felt:

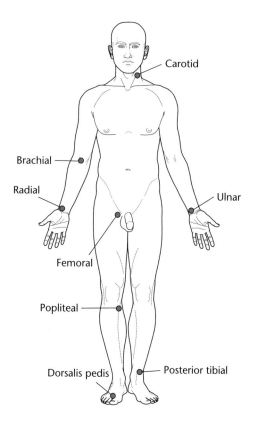

ABNORMAL RATE

INCREASED RATE

Tachycardia

Response to an increased
need for circulating oxygen:
A raised metabolic rate
- Exercise
- Fever
- Hyperthyroidism
- Stress

A diminished flow of
circulating oxygen:
- Haemorrhage
- Heart failure
- Arrhythmias

Disorders of the pumping
mechanism:
- Atrial tachycardia
- Junctional tachycardia
- Supraventricular tachycardia
- Ventricular tachycardia

Drugs, including:
- Salbutamol
- Captopril

DECREASED RATE

Bradycardia

Response to a decreased
need for circulating oxygen:
A lowered metabolic rate
- The elderly
- Athletes, at rest
- Hypothyroidism
- Hypothermia

Disorders of the pumping
mechanism:
- Heart block

Raised intercranial pressure

Drugs, including:
- Beta-blockers
- Cimetidine

ABSENCE OF PERIPHERAL PULSES

Obstruction of the circulating blood above site of pulse:
- Thrombus
- Embolus
- Tight bandaging
- Constriction from plaster of Paris splint
- Heart has stopped pumping

ABNORMAL CHARACTERISTICS

ABNORMAL RHYTHMS

Sinus arrhythmia
Increased rate on inspiration, slows on expiration.

– A normal pattern; does not indicate disease

Irregular beats or extra beats.

– Atrial fibrillation
  Ectopic beats
  Heart block

Alternating pulse
Weak and strong alternating beats, in a regular rhythm.

– Tachycardia
  Severe myocardial failure

Pulsus bisferiens
The pulse has a double rhythm to each beat.

– Disorders preventing the proper emptying of the left ventricle

VARIATION IN VOLUME

Increase in pulse volume
Signifies attempted increase in cardiac output; can be a compensation mechanism.

– Fever
  Thyrotoxicosis
  Bradycardia
  Aortic valve incompetence

Decrease in pulse volume
Decreased pressure with each beat.

– Tachycardia
  Cardiac failure
  Obstruction to cardiac blood flow
  Hypothermia

Paradoxical pulse
The pulse varies in volume with each respiration.
A normal occurrence especially in children.
Becomes abnormal when the change in volume becomes exaggerated.

– Asthma
  Pericardial effusion
  Constructive pericarditis

VISIBLE CAROTID PULSE

Often seen in ageing women, when tissues fail to support the carotid artery and it begins to 'kink'. Also seen in aneurysms, hypertension and conditions causing an increased cardiac output.

ASSOCIATED INVESTIGATIONS

		Related pages
Skin colour	The presence of central cyanosis, peripheral cyanosis or pallor will indicate a failing circulation and oxygen supply to tissues. The skin will become clammy to touch as the skin vasoconstricts in an attempt to support oxygenation of vital organs.	272
Apical beat	This direct way of counting heart beats is a more appropriate method for measuring the heart rate of neonates and young babies. Simultaneous counting of the apical beat and the radial pulse will recognise a deficit between the count taken of the heart rate and the number of beats reaching the peripheral pulses.	10
Blood pressure	Heart rate and cardiac volume are components of the system that controls the blood pressure. Alterations in the pulse will stimulate compensatory mechanisms to make adjustments. This allows the blood pressure to remain within normal limits.	17
Respirations	The pulse rate will alter according to the body's need for oxygen. Respiration rates also change on the same basis. Breathlessness and cough can also be significant.	129
Haemoglobin values	Severe anaemia will increase the work of the heart. The depleted availability of haemoglobin will reduce the quantity of oxygen that can be carried for tissue oxygenation.	38
Auscultation	Examination with a stethoscope to detect abnormalities of the pumping mechanism of the heart.	
Temperature	Temperature may rise in response to cardiac damage or inflammatory cardiac disorder.	4
Oedema	Oedematous legs, or oedema seen at the lowest gravitational point, according to the position of the patient. The oedema shows indentations or 'pits' when superficial pressure is applied – a sign of congestive cardiac failure.	283
Electrocardiogram	The examination of the electrical impulses that stimulate the heart to beat.	24
Scanning and imaging techniques	These give clear pictures of the heart while it is at work. They therefore identify points of dysfunction that impede the efficiency of the heart. ■ Echogram ■ Nuclear imaging	297

CONSIDERATIONS FOR CARE

The proper assessment of a pulse can be difficult. Physical effort prior to the examination and the stresses associated with health checks have an immediate effect on the pulse rate. If it is not essential that the pulse be taken immediately, the nurse should delay taking the pulse until the patient appears rested and at ease.

Young children may dislike having their hand held in one position by a person that they do not know. It can be upsetting and frightening for them. A less distressing pulse to use, when the child is awake, is the temporal pulse, taken from behind the child as they cuddle into their parents.

The radial pulse may be weak in neonates and young babies. The apical beat should be taken in place of the peripheral pulse in these circumstances.

The pulse rate is frequently checked during the acute phase of treatment or disease, i.e. post-operatively. The nurse must not rely on the pulse rate alone as an indication of well-being. The heart and circulation can use compensating mechanisms to maintain stability even when the patient's condition is deteriorating. Respirations, skin colour and texture, and the patient's demeanour should all be taken into consideration each time the pulse is taken.

The peripheral pulses may become absent as the blood circulation fails. The absence of the carotid pulse signals cardiac arrest. Resuscitation procedures should then be initiated if appropriate.

REFERENCE RANGE

Adult: 120/80 mmHg

Child: ranges,   80–110/45–65 mmHg

Neonate: ranges,   65–95/30–60 mmHg   – A mean measurement is calculated:

$$\frac{\text{Systolic pressure} - \text{diastolic pressure}}{3} + \text{diastolic pressure} = \text{mean blood pressure}$$

PROCEDURE

A sphygmomanometer:
- Manual + stethoscope
- Electronic.

Many devices for measuring blood pressure are now available. Accurate recordings depend on the user receiving proper instruction prior to operating the machines.
- The patient's arm must be comfortable and well supported throughout the procedure.
- Stress and activity will cause the blood pressure to rise.
- Clothing must not constrict the limb used to take the blood pressure.
- When a patient needs regular blood pressure monitoring, the same size cuff must be used each time.
- Blood pressures taken on a crying, wriggling child will be inaccurate and distressing to the child, parent and nurse. Give comfort, assurance and distraction.
- Blood pressure should not be taken on an arm with an intravenous infusion in progress. The pressure may dislodge the cannula.

PURPOSE

To measure the force exerted by blood against the walls of arterial blood vessels.

The measurement taken has two parts:
- The highest number is the pressure of blood in the arteries when the ventricles of the heart are contracting – the systolic pressure.
- The lowest number is the pressure of blood in the arteries when the ventricles are at rest – the diastolic pressure.

The blood pressure depends on:

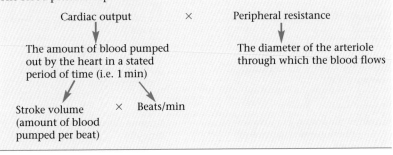

Cardiac output   ×   Peripheral resistance

The amount of blood pumped out by the heart in a stated period of time (i.e. 1 min)

The diameter of the arteriole through which the blood flows

Stroke volume × Beats/min
(amount of blood pumped per beat)

Changes in any part of this system will alter the recorded blood pressure, although compensatory mechanisms will attempt to keep the blood pressure within normal limits.

NORMAL PHYSIOLOGY

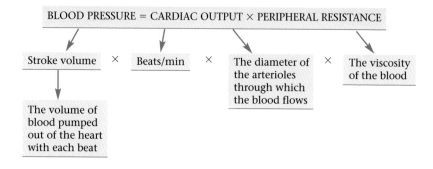

BLOOD PRESSURE = CARDIAC OUTPUT × PERIPHERAL RESISTANCE

| Stroke volume | × | Beats/min | × | The diameter of the arterioles through which the blood flows | × | The viscosity of the blood |

The volume of blood pumped out of the heart with each beat

The maintenance of a normal blood pressure relies on the balance and the adjustment of the systems that modify the factors that produce a cardiac output and the peripheral resistance.

The blood pressure is monitored by:

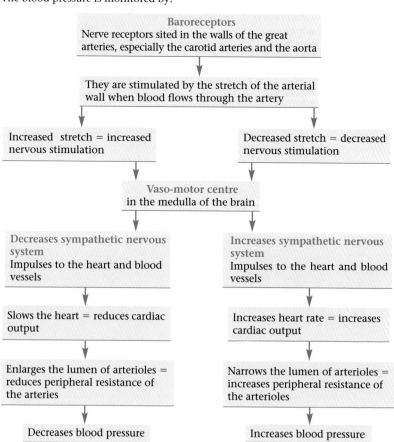

Baroreceptors
Nerve receptors sited in the walls of the great arteries, especially the carotid arteries and the aorta

They are stimulated by the stretch of the arterial wall when blood flows through the artery

Increased stretch = increased nervous stimulation

Decreased stretch = decreased nervous stimulation

Vaso-motor centre
in the medulla of the brain

Decreases sympathetic nervous system
Impulses to the heart and blood vessels

Increases sympathetic nervous system
Impulses to the heart and blood vessels

Slows the heart = reduces cardiac output

Increases heart rate = increases cardiac output

Enlarges the lumen of arterioles = reduces peripheral resistance of the arteries

Narrows the lumen of arterioles = increases peripheral resistance of the arterioles

Decreases blood pressure

Increases blood pressure

ALTERED VALUES

RAISED BLOOD PRESSURE	LOW BLOOD PRESSURE
Hypertension	**Hypotension**

Stroke volume increased
- Increase in blood volume
- Increase in extracellular fluid retention
- Obesity
- Adrenal tumour releasing aldosterone increases fluid retention by kidneys, causing blood volume to rise
- Pre-eclampsia in pregnancy

Stroke volume decreased
- Decrease in blood volume
- Hypovolaemic shock
- Cardiogenic shock
- Septic shock
- Anaphylactic shock
- Neurogenic shock
- Sodium deficiency

Increase in heart rate
Stimulation of the sympathetic nervous system
- Anxiety
- Pain
- Excitement
- Exercise
- Fever

Decrease in heart rate
Decreased activity of the sympathetic nervous system
- Bradycardia

Narrowing of the arteriole lumen through which blood flows
- Arteriosclerosis
- Atheroma
- Cold
- Diseased ischaemic kidneys secreting renin

Dilation of the arteriole lumen through which blood flows
- Warmth

Increase in blood viscosity
- Polycythaemia

Decrease in blood viscosity
- Reduction in number of red cells

Essential hypertension
No cause identified

Drugs, including:
- Oral contraceptives with oestrogen
- Non-steroidal anti-inflammatory drugs
- Corticosteroids

Drugs, including:
- Lidocaine
- Enoximone

ADJUSTMENT MECHANISMS

RENAL – BODY FLUID CONTROL

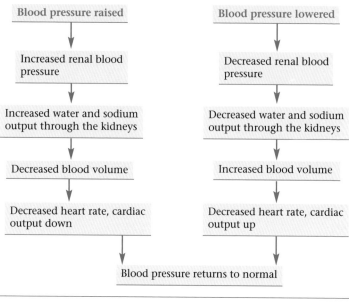

Blood pressure raised

↓

Increased renal blood pressure

↓

Increased water and sodium output through the kidneys

↓

Decreased blood volume

↓

Decreased heart rate, cardiac output down

Blood pressure lowered

↓

Decreased renal blood pressure

↓

Decreased water and sodium output through the kidneys

↓

Increased blood volume

↓

Decreased heart rate, cardiac output up

Blood pressure returns to normal

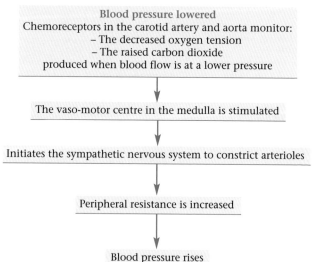

Blood pressure lowered
Chemoreceptors in the carotid artery and aorta monitor:
– The decreased oxygen tension
– The raised carbon dioxide
produced when blood flow is at a lower pressure

↓

The vaso-motor centre in the medulla is stimulated

↓

Initiates the sympathetic nervous system to constrict arterioles

↓

Peripheral resistance is increased

↓

Blood pressure rises

RENIN–ANGIOTENSIN MECHANISM

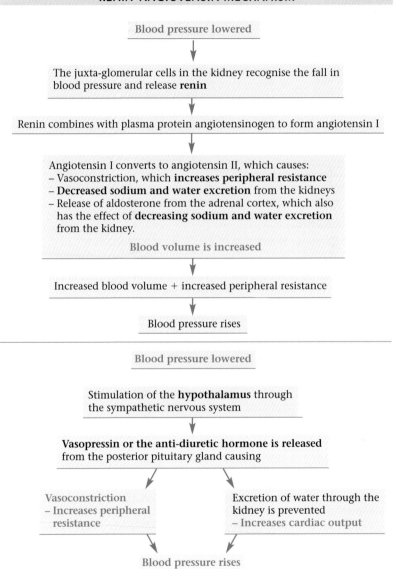

Blood pressure lowered

↓

The juxta-glomerular cells in the kidney recognise the fall in blood pressure and release **renin**

↓

Renin combines with plasma protein angiotensinogen to form angiotensin I

↓

Angiotensin I converts to angiotensin II, which causes:
– Vasoconstriction, which **increases peripheral resistance**
– **Decreased sodium and water excretion** from the kidneys
– Release of aldosterone from the adrenal cortex, which also has the effect of **decreasing sodium and water excretion** from the kidney.

Blood volume is increased

↓

Increased blood volume + increased peripheral resistance

↓

Blood pressure rises

Blood pressure lowered

Stimulation of the **hypothalamus** through the sympathetic nervous system

↓

Vasopressin or the anti-diuretic hormone is released from the posterior pituitary gland causing

Vasoconstriction
– Increases peripheral resistance

Excretion of water through the kidney is prevented
– Increases cardiac output

Blood pressure rises

ASSOCIATED INVESTIGATIONS

		Related pages
Pulse	Heart rate is part of the cardiac output calculation.	9
Respirations	Increased: ■ When sympathetic nervous system stimulated, e.g. stress, anxiety ■ In hypoxic states, e.g. reduced blood volume.	129
Skin temperature, skin colour, clammy or dry	Assess the state of peripheral vasodilation or vasoconstriction.	269
Colour of mucous membranes	Dark red in polycythaemia. Light red in low red blood cell count.	34
Lying and standing blood pressure for postural hypotension	Autonomic reflexes counter the effect of gravity on blood when altering body position from lying to standing. Vasoconstriction maintains an adequate blood supply to the brain. This mechanisms is tested by: ■ Taking the blood pressure after the patient has been lying quietly for some minutes; early morning is the best time for this. ■ Ask or help the patient to stand; retake the blood pressure. ■ Note if there is a difference in the two readings.	17
Urinalysis	Test for the presence of protein as an indication of renal disease.	189
Urea, creatinine	Tests of renal function.	119
Chest X-ray	May show cardiac enlargement, abnormalities of the large vessels.	295
Electrocardiogram	Test for presence of cardiac disease.	24

CONSIDERATIONS FOR CARE

RAISED BLOOD PRESSURE (HYPERTENSION)

Staff should provide a relaxing environment that allows the patient to feel comfortable and secure when coming to the clinic or hospital for their blood pressure to be monitored.

The control of hypertension will probably continue for the rest of the patient's life. These patients will need to feel supported by the staff, when attempting to alter long-standing habits and patterns that may have contributed to their hypertension. Advice will only be accepted by the patient when they trust the counsellor.

To comply with the requirements of long-term medication is often difficult. Explanation of the benefits and effects of the drugs will be needed, and warnings of possible side-effects. If the patient reports difficulties with the medication, alternative drugs must be examined as the patient may not continue the therapy if it makes them feel worse than the original condition being treated.

Dietary advice should be available if the patient is overweight. Strategies to limit alcohol intake and cigarette smoking must be offered.

The patient's own way of dealing with stress must be explored.

LOWERED BLOOD PRESSURE (HYPOTENSION)

When hypotension, or sudden episodes of hypotension, present a prolonged problem, care must be taken when getting out of bed or up from a chair. Dizziness and fainting may be a problem.

Hot baths, producing vasodilation, will cause dizziness when the patient stands to get out.

Acute shock will produce a fall in blood pressure. This will occur with the failure of the adjustment mechanisms that keep the blood pressure within normal limits under abnormal circumstances.

- Lie the patient flat to aid blood flow to the brain.
- If possible, talk to the patient, and offer assurance.
- Summon medical help, to correct the cause of the shocked condition.
- Regularly monitor the temperature, pulse, respirations and blood pressure.
- Note changes in skin colour, temperature and degree of dryness.
- Monitor the urinary output as an indication of renal function and cardiac output.
- Note any change in consciousness.

NORMAL MEASUREMENT

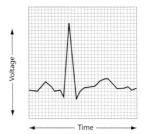

PROCEDURE

Sensors and leads attached to an electrocardiogram monitor are fastened to the body.

The position and number of leads will depend on the type of electrocardiogram monitor used.

The monitor registers the electrical impulses passing through the myocardium of the heart.

A printed record is made of these electrical tracings.

The sensors and the skin must be in close, secure contact. An electrode gel is applied between the sensor and the skin to improve the conduction of electrical impulses between the skin and the sensor.

When explaining the procedure, assure the patient that the electricity recorded is coming *from* their body to the machine.

The patient needs to lie still while the recording is taken.

For the comfort of the patient, remove the gel properly from the skin after the recording.

PURPOSE

To make a visual recording of the electrical impulses passing through the cells of the myocardium. From this, the rate, rhythm and strength of each heart beat can be assessed.

A predetermined series of events generates a normal heart beat.

These events are stimulated by the conduction of electrical action potentials through the heart muscle, causing the cells of the myocardium to contract.

They follow established pathways through the myocardium.

The effect of the electrical impulse is to produce rhythmic, alternating contractions of the atria and the ventricles.

One set of atrial and ventricular contractions producing a single heart beat is termed the 'cardiac cycle'.

The electrocardiogram records the electrical activity in the heart on graph paper.

The horizontal lines on the graph paper record the travelling time of electrical impulses through each phase of the cardiac cycle.

The vertical lines measure the voltage of the electrical stimulus.

The normal heart beat will set a standard tracing, depicting electrical pathways, timing and voltage.

This normal tracing is then used as a model for comparison.

NORMAL PHYSIOLOGY

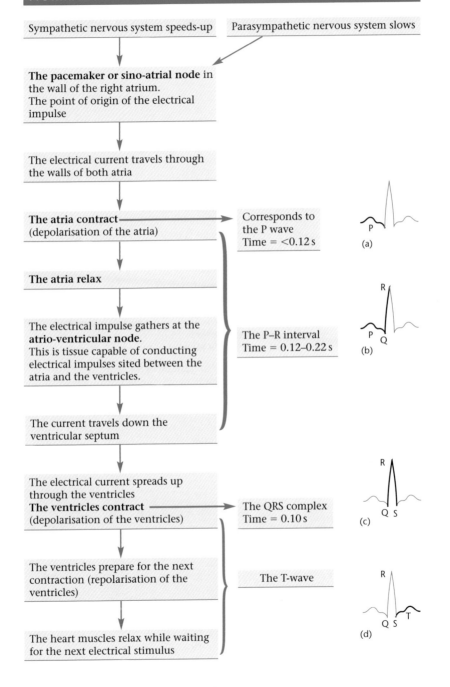

Sympathetic nervous system speeds-up

Parasympathetic nervous system slows

The pacemaker or sino-atrial node in the wall of the right atrium.
The point of origin of the electrical impulse

The electrical current travels through the walls of both atria

The atria contract
(depolarisation of the atria)

Corresponds to the P wave
Time = <0.12 s

(a)

The atria relax

The electrical impulse gathers at the **atrio-ventricular node**.
This is tissue capable of conducting electrical impulses sited between the atria and the ventricles.

The P–R interval
Time = 0.12–0.22 s

(b)

The current travels down the ventricular septum

The electrical current spreads up through the ventricles
The ventricles contract
(depolarisation of the ventricles)

The QRS complex
Time = 0.10 s

(c)

The ventricles prepare for the next contraction (repolarisation of the ventricles)

The T-wave

(d)

The heart muscles relax while waiting for the next electrical stimulus

ABNORMAL TRACINGS

Specialist knowledge is needed to interpret the fine variations of electrocardiograph recordings.

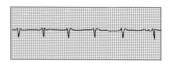

Normal sinus rhythm

The examples given are the more obvious deviations from normal.

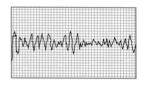

Asystole:
– An absence of electrical activity within the heart muscle

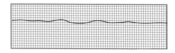

Ventricular fibrillation:
– The ventricular motion is rapid and weak
– The heart is no longer pumping blood
– Cardiac resuscitation is necessary

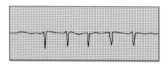

Atrioventricular block:
– The electrical impulses are blocked between the atria and the ventricles. Several types occur, for example:
– The PR interval is prolonged

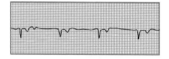

– A partial heart block showing two P waves before each QRS complex

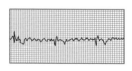

Atrial flutter

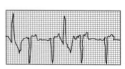

Ventricular ectopic beats

ASSOCIATED INVESTIGATIONS

		Related pages
Pulse	An assessment of the rate, rhythm and volume of heart beats.	9
Blood pressure	The cardiac output is a major factor in the control of blood pressure.	17
Chest X-ray	Shows the size and shape of the heart.	295
Exercise electrocardiography	Shows the response of the heart to exercise. The recording is taken as the patient exercises. The point at which changes occurred can then be marked.	
24-hour ambulatory taped electrocardiography	A method of recording intermittent changes in cardiac electrical conductivity. This is useful when the stimulus that provokes the onset of arrhythmias can not be simulated.	
Auscultation of the heart	Examination of the heart using a stethoscope, to detect abnormalities of the pumping mechanism.	
Cardiac enzymes	A pattern of changing values, over time, of the enzymes creatine phosphokinase (CPK) , aspartate aminotransferase (AST) and lactate dehydrogenase (LDH) can indicate myocardial damage.	
Echocardiography	This test is an ultrasound technique. It displays moving pictures of the heart onto a screen. It shows the size, structure and motion of the heart, from which abnormalities can be recognised.	298
Nuclear imaging techniques ■ Thallium-201 imaging	The use of radioactive markers to give accurate positioning of a myocardial infarction.	297
Cardiac catheterisation	An invasive technique. Using a route through the venous system, a catheter is introduced into the heart and main blood vessels around the heart. Purposes: ■ Pressure measurements can be taken. ■ Blood samples are withdrawn from different areas of the heart to measure oxygen and metabolite levels. ■ Cardiac angiography. Radio-opaque dye is introduced through the catheter to give X-ray pictures of the cardiac chambers and blood vessels.	

CENTRAL VENOUS PRESSURE

REFERENCE RANGE

3–8 cm of water or 2–6 mmHg

PROCEDURE

A three-way fluid-filled system connects a bag of infusion fluid, a manometer or electrical transducer, and a long catheter that has its tip in the superior vena cava. Following the proper positioning of the patient, the three-way tap can be manipulated until the manometer, or electric transducer, will record the pressure of blood in the right atrium of the heart. Instruction is essential before implementing this procedure, as an incorrect technique can introduce air into the system. This is potentially dangerous to the patient.

Using a peripheral vein as an entry site, the catheter is threaded through a venous channel until the catheter tip rests in the superior vena cava. The catheter must be attached securely to the skin. This is a sterile procedure.

The reference point for measurement should be marked on the skin.

The patient must lie at the same angle to the manometer each time the measurement is taken.

PURPOSE

To measure the pressure at which the blood enters the right atrium of the heart. Under normal circumstances, blood is at atmospheric pressure at this point, having no other physiological forces on its flow.

The central venous pressure monitors:
- The volume of blood in the venous system
- The efficiency of the right ventricle of the heart
- The tone held by the venous walls.

Changes in any one of these three factors will cause an altered central venous pressure recording.

Central venous pressure is most often used to monitor large changes in blood volume:
- Hypervolaemia will cause the central venous pressure to rise
- Hypovolaemia will cause the central venous pressure to fall.

Changes in central venous pressure will also assess the efficiency of the right side of the heart to expel venous blood into the pulmonary artery.

It is also used to assess the ability of the right atrium to deal with blood entering the heart.

NORMAL PHYSIOLOGY

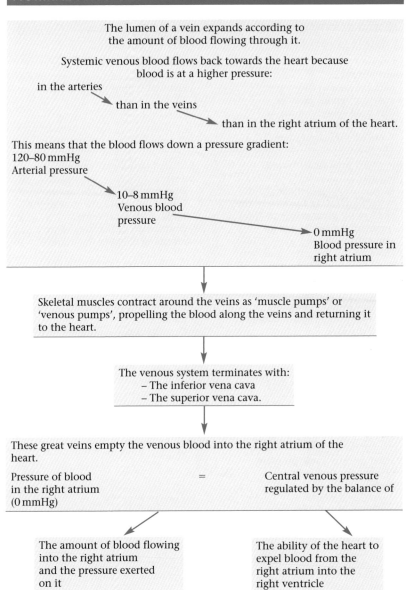

The lumen of a vein expands according to the amount of blood flowing through it.

Systemic venous blood flows back towards the heart because blood is at a higher pressure:

in the arteries

than in the veins

than in the right atrium of the heart.

This means that the blood flows down a pressure gradient:
120–80 mmHg
Arterial pressure

10–8 mmHg
Venous blood
pressure

0 mmHg
Blood pressure in
right atrium

Skeletal muscles contract around the veins as 'muscle pumps' or 'venous pumps', propelling the blood along the veins and returning it to the heart.

The venous system terminates with:
– The inferior vena cava
– The superior vena cava.

These great veins empty the venous blood into the right atrium of the heart.

| Pressure of blood in the right atrium (0 mmHg) | = | Central venous pressure regulated by the balance of |

The amount of blood flowing into the right atrium and the pressure exerted on it

The ability of the heart to expel blood from the right atrium into the right ventricle

ALTERED VALUES

RAISED CENTRAL VENOUS PRESSURE

Increased pressure in the right atrium
- Back pressure in the systemic venous pressure
- Increased venous return
- Decreased cardiac output
- Reduced arterial pressure

Increased peripheral venous pressure
- Increased sympathetic nervous system increasing the tone of the walls of the great veins
- Increased contraction of all skeletal muscles
- Dilatation of the arteries allows rapid blood flow from the arteries to the veins

Increased blood volume
- Excessive transfusion of fluids
- Renal disease

Decreased ability of the heart to pump
- Heart failure
- Myocardial infarction
- Valvular heart disease
- Fluid collection within the pericardium

Raised intrathoracic pressure
- Respiratory disease
- Pleural effusions

LOWERED CENTRAL VENOUS PRESSURE

Reduced pressure in the right atrium
- Reduced venous return of blood

Reduced peripheral venous pressure
- Decreased sympathetic nervous system decreasing the tone of the walls of the great veins
- Obstruction of the large veins returning blood to the heart

Decreased blood volume
- Haemorrhage
- Dehydration

Increased ability of the heart to pump

ASSOCIATED INVESTIGATIONS

		Related pages
Distension of neck veins	Neck veins are not normally distended. As the central venous pressure rises the neck veins begin to protrude. When the central venous pressure is very high the neck veins protrude and a pulse becomes evident.	
Fluid input and output chart	The infusion of intravenous fluid is part of the central venous pressure recording.	
Temperature	To detect the development of infection along the catheter.	4
Pulse and blood pressure	To regularly assess cardiac and circulatory function.	9, 17
Electrocardiogram	An assessment of the rate, rhythm and strength of the heart beat.	24

CONSIDERATIONS FOR CARE

Abnormally raised or lowered central venous pressure measurements will indicate a distressed cardiac or circulatory system.

Elements of care will depend on the treatment of the underlying condition.

Expectations of mobility and self-care will be modified by the severity of the disorder and the limitations of being attached to the central venous pressure line and equipment.

Restricted movement from the bed is possible, but the central venous pressure lines must not be stretched or disconnected. Extreme care is needed when helping the patient on to a commode or chair.

The patient will probably need repositioning to realign the reference points of measurement.

If moving is difficult or painful for the patient, this time should also be used to complete all the other necessary care.

This will ensure that the patient has minimal disturbance between each reading and their rest and sleep are not disturbed unnecessarily.

The position of the catheter tip at the entrance of the right atria makes it imperative that infection does not enter the line.

Aseptic precautions must be taken:
- At the point of its insertion into the skin
- With all fluids entering the line.

The line must be checked regularly for air pockets.

The line is kept patent by the constant flow of infusion fluid.

An accurate input and output fluid chart must be maintained as:
- A record of the infused intravenous fluid must be kept
- The combined amounts of the intravenous fluid and oral fluids must be compared to the urine output
- The combined fluid intake and output must be assessed against changes in the central venous pressure measurement.

The patient with respiratory disease who likes to remain in an upright position may be distressed by the lying or inclined position needed to measure the central venous pressure.

Blood is routinely taken for testing using the techniques of venepuncture, heel prick or finger-tip prick. Arterial blood is used for blood gas analysis.

All blood-taking techniques must be carried out under the terms of local policy. This will designate the staff who are authorised to take blood and set the basis for practical procedure.

Some considerations always apply:
- The patient must be given an explanation of the procedure and the reason why it is necessary.
- The patient must be informed of the time when the results of the test will be available and how they will be able to obtain them.
- Staff must be careful to avoid coming into direct contact with the patient's blood or pricking themselves with a contaminated needle.
- Aseptic technique must always be used when taking a blood sample.
- The patient should be made as comfortable as possible. The extended arm must be kept straight and well supported.
- A child will need constant reassurance, preferably by its mother. Toys, games and rewards may help.
- If an intravenous infusion is in progress, take the blood sample from the opposite arm, as the infusion fluid may affect the results.
- Prolonged use of the tourniquet will cause intravascular fluid to move into surrounding tissues. If this happens, the blood sample will not be accurate and false results will occur.
- Avoid squeezing too hard when using the heel prick technique. It is painful and inaccurate results will occur (reason as above).
- Invert rather than shake specimens to mix. This will prevent the blood sample becoming haemolysed.
- Apply firm and prolonged pressure to the puncture site to avoid haematoma formation.
- When considering blood results, remember that they can be modified by many things, e.g. drugs, exercise, posture, diurnal patterns and genetic make-up.
- The accuracy of the results may be time critical. Some blood test results become meaningless if a time limit is allowed to lapse before the analysis.

RED BLOOD CELLS

RED BLOOD CELL OR ERYTHROCYTE COUNT

REFERENCE RANGE

Adult: Male: 4.5–6.0×10^{12}/litre
              Female: 3.9–5.1×10^{12}/litre

Child: 4.2–5.4×10^{12}/litre

Neonate: 4.5–5.0×10^{12}/litre

PROCEDURE

Venepuncture.

CONTAINER

The specimen container used in this unit is:

PURPOSE

To ensure that the red blood cell count is within normal limits.

The red blood cell or erythrocyte contains haemoglobin, the transport molecule that picks up and carries oxygen around the blood circulation.

The bi-concave shape of this un-nucleated cell allows the maximum surface area for oxygen to transfer across the red blood cell wall.

This transfer occurs when:
- Oxygen is picked up from inspired air by the haemoglobin in the arterial blood capillaries within the alveoli of the lungs.
- Oxygen is taken from the circulating haemoglobin, by the cells of the body, to provide energy for metabolic function.

The red blood cell also contains carbonic anhydrase. This enzyme speeds up the reaction between carbon dioxide and water, hastening the removal of carbon dioxide from the tissues.

The red blood cells act as an acid–base buffer, to keep the pH of the blood at 7.4.

A lowered red blood cell count will lower the available oxygen-carrying capacity of the blood. Hypoxia stimulates the mechanism that stimulates bone marrow to manufacture more red blood cells.

A raised red blood cell count increases the oxygen-carrying capacity of the blood. A raised red cell count is able to compensate when the amount of inspired oxygen is reduced. The increased number of cells will provide the additional transport molecules to accept and circulate all the available oxygen that reaches the alveoli.

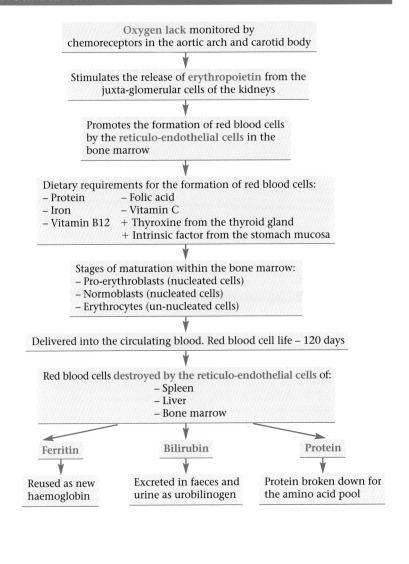

Oxygen lack monitored by
chemoreceptors in the aortic arch and carotid body

Stimulates the release of erythropoietin from the
juxta-glomerular cells of the kidneys

Promotes the formation of red blood cells
by the reticulo-endothelial cells in the
bone marrow

Dietary requirements for the formation of red blood cells:
– Protein   – Folic acid
– Iron   – Vitamin C
– Vitamin B12   + Thyroxine from the thyroid gland
                + Intrinsic factor from the stomach mucosa

Stages of maturation within the bone marrow:
– Pro-erythroblasts (nucleated cells)
– Normoblasts (nucleated cells)
– Erythrocytes (un-nucleated cells)

Delivered into the circulating blood. Red blood cell life – 120 days

Red blood cells destroyed by the reticulo-endothelial cells of:
– Spleen
– Liver
– Bone marrow

Ferritin

Bilirubin

Protein

Reused as new
haemoglobin

Excreted in faeces and
urine as urobilinogen

Protein broken down for
the amino acid pool

ALTERED VALUES

RAISED VALUES

Erythrocytosis
Reaction to prolonged depletion
of oxygen in the blood
– Pulmonary disease
– Heart disease
– High altitude

Decreased blood flow to
kidneys
– Shock

Increased production of
erythropoietin
– Renal cysts
– Some renal tumours

Polycythaemia
– Overactive reticulo-
  endothelial system
– Smoking

Decrease in circulating fluid
volume
– Burns
– Dehydration
– Diarrhoea

LOWERED VALUES

Renal failure
Surgical removal of kidney

Deficiency anaemia
– Hypothyroidism
– Lack of dietary
  requirements
– Failure to produce
  intrinsic factor

Pernicious anaemia

Aplastic anaemia
– Degeneration of
  bone marrow

Following haemorrhage
– Replacement fluids to
  restore blood volume will
  reduce the number of red
  cells per ml of blood

Haemolytic anaemia
Red blood cell destruction rate
exceeds manufacture rate
– Thalassaemia
– Sickle cell anaemia

ASSOCIATED INVESTIGATIONS

		Related pages
Pulse	The pulse increases when the oxygen-carrying component of the blood is reduced.	9
Respirations	The rate of respirations increases when the oxygen-carrying capacity of the blood is reduced.	129
Blood pressure	A very low red blood cell count, if left untreated, will cause the heart to fail. A reflection of this is a lowered blood pressure. Excessive numbers of red blood cells will increase blood viscosity and raise the blood pressure.	17
Haemoglobin	To assess the haemoglobin content of the red blood cells.	38
Serum iron	Iron bound to the transport protein transferrin, in the plasma.	
Mean corpuscular volume (MCV)	Helps when differentiating anaemias. Microcytosis – a reduced cell diameter. Macrocytosis – an enlarged cell diameter.	
Mean corpuscular haemoglobin concentration (MCHC)	The concentration of haemoglobin expressed as a proportion of the red cell content of the blood.	
Total iron binding capacity	This measures the amount of iron that the blood is capable of transporting, if all the iron binding sites were in use.	
Haematocrit or packed cell volume (PCV)	The measurement of the red blood cell content, expressed as a percentage of the total volume of blood.	
Erythrocyte sedimentation rate (ESR)	The measured amount of erythrocytes that settle at the bottom of a tube of blood over a set period of time.	43
A blood film	The microscopic examination of the red blood cells.	
Bone marrow puncture	The examination of the development of the red blood cell. Also the development of the white blood cells and platelets.	71
Glucose-6-phosphate dehydrogenase screen	An enzyme found in the red blood cell. A deficiency of this enzyme will reduce the life span of the red blood cell and be a cause of a haemolytic anaemia.	
Schilling test	Vitamin B12, an essential for red blood cell production is absorbed from the ileum, in the presence of intrinsic factor secreted from the stomach. A Schilling test will determine whether a lack of vitamin B12 is due to a lack of secreted intrinsic factor or small intestine malabsorption.	

REFERENCE RANGE

Adult: Male: 13–18 g/dl
        Female: 11.5–15.5 g/dl

Child: Boys: 14 g/dl
        Girls: 13.8 g/dl

Neonate: 16.6 g/dl

The value falls to 11 g/dl blood at age 3 months and then gradually rises to standard children's values.

PROCEDURE

Venepuncture.

Prolonged use of tourniquet will raise the haemoglobin level.

CONTAINER

The specimen container used in this unit is:

PURPOSE

To determine the amount of haemoglobin available in the red blood cells for oxygen transport.

Haemoglobin is an iron-containing molecule found in red blood cells. It has the ability to combine with and transport oxygen.

Oxygen from inspired air is picked up by haemoglobin as the red cells pass through the pulmonary capillary blood vessels. Haemoglobin then transports the oxygen in the circulating blood. The haemoglobin gives up the oxygen, which passes across the arterial capillary walls, to enter cells. Oxygen is used by cells for energy production. It is this energy that provides power for cell metabolism and enables the cell to fulfil its function.

A *lack* of haemoglobin would result in a reduced oxygen supply to cells; a reduced supply of fuel for cell metabolism.

A *raised* haemoglobin level would indicate a blood picture with a raised number of red blood cells, as there is a limit to the amount of haemoglobin that each red cell can carry.

When measured, the iron binding capacity of the blood will rise when an iron deficiency anaemia diminishes the amount of iron needing transport around the body. It will fall when iron is plentiful and filling all available sites.

Iron present in food.

↓

Iron absorbed by the upper small intestine, in the presence of vitamin C.

The amount of iron absorbed = the amount needed for haemoglobin manufacture.

The rest is excreted.

Absorbed iron becomes attached to a protein for transport in plasma and becomes transferrin.

↓

This is taken to:
– Bone marrow for the manufacture of haemoglobin
– Liver, spleen and bone marrow for storage as ferritin.

↓

Haemoglobin is carried in the red blood cells for the transport of oxygen.

↓

Haemoglobin is released when the red blood cell is destroyed (120 days).

↓

The molecule splits into haem and the protein globin.

Haem
Ferritin removed and stored for reuse.
Rest of molecule converted to bilirubin and biliverdin.

↓

Taken to the liver and enters the small intestine through the bile duct.

↓

Excreted in the stool or urine as urobilinogen.

Globin
Protein broken down into amino acids.

↓

Returned to amino acid pool for reuse.

ALTERED VALUES

RAISED VALUES	REDUCED VALUES
	Anaemia
	Dietary deficiencies – Iron-deficiency anaemia – Vitamin C deficiency
	Reduced iron absorption – Inadequate levels of transferrin

Excessive production
of red blood cells
– Polycythaemia
– Hypoxia from:
  – Pulmonary disease
  – Congenital heart
    disease
  – High altitudes
	Reduced number of
	manufactured red blood
	cells
	– Pernicious anaemia
	– Underactive thyroid
	– Bone marrow disease
	  – Leukaemia
	  – Aplastic anaemia

	Following haemorrhage acute or chronic
	Excessive breakdown of red blood cells – Haemolytic anaemia – Haemolytic disease of the newborn
Loss of circulating fluid volume – Severe burns – Lack of oral fluids – Diarrhoea – Vomiting	Expanded plasma volume – Pregnancy – Excessive intravenous therapy
	Drugs, including: – Cytotoxic drugs

ASSOCIATED INVESTIGATIONS

		Related pages
Pulse	Haemoglobin carries oxygen to cells. The pulse rate increases when the supply of oxygen is reduced.	9
Blood pressure	Prolonged severe anaemia can become a cause of heart failure.	17
Mean corpuscular volume	The size of the red cell will vary according to the condition causing the anaemia.	
Mean corpuscular haemoglobin concentration (MCHC)	The red blood cells become hypochromic or pale when their haemoglobin concentration is reduced.	
Mean corpuscular haemoglobin (MCH)	This measures the weight of the red blood cell. The cell weight increases with the amount of haemoglobin present.	
Red blood cell platelet count	This will vary with: ■ Haemorrhage ■ Disordered blood cell production in the bone marrow.	34 63
Serum ferritin	An indicator of the amount of iron stored for use.	
Serum iron	The amount of iron available for storage and use.	
Total iron binding capacity	The number of binding sites available to iron in the blood for transport in the blood: transferrin and other plasma proteins.	
Haematocrit or packed cell volume (PCV)	The volume of red blood cells, expressed as a percentage of the circulating blood.	
The degree of redness of the mucous membranes	The colour of the mucous membranes reflects the haemoglobin content of the red blood cell, from the pallor of anaemia to the dusky red of polycythaemia.	
Cord blood of neonate taken at birth	This allows detection of rhesus incompatibility if the tests show: ■ Low haemoglobin ■ Raised bilirubin ■ Positive Coombs' test, indicating the presence of antibodies on the red blood cells.	

RED BLOOD CELL COUNT AND HAEMOGLOBIN VALUES

CONSIDERATIONS FOR CARE

RAISED RED BLOOD CELL COUNT
RAISED HAEMOGLOBIN LEVELS

A raised number of circulating red blood cells will increase the viscosity of the blood. This can lead to:
- Raised blood pressure
- Headache
- Dizziness
- Tinnitus.

The increased haemoglobin value will give the patient's mucous membranes a dark red appearance.

When polycythaemia is present, a volume of blood may be drawn off by venesection to reduce the discomfort felt by the patient.

Foods with a high iron content should be avoided.

LOW RED BLOOD CELL COUNT
LOW HAEMOGLOBIN LEVELS

These conditions will lower the oxygen supply to the cells of the body.

The amount of debility that this brings will depend on the cause and severity of the anaemia. The following description of potential patient problems must be considered according to the degree of haemoglobin depletion:
- Reduced circulating haemoglobin will give the patient a pallor of the mucous membranes.
- A diminished supply of oxygen to fuel cell metabolism will cause:
  - Lethargy
  - Tachycardia, palpitations
  - Breathlessness on exertion
  - Dizziness, headache.
- When anaemia is caused by the increased destruction of red blood cells, the increased amount of the breakdown product bilirubin may cause jaundice.
- Nursing care must be sensitive to the degree of debility felt by the patient. Walking and exercise may be exhausting, especially if there is an underlying cardiac or respiratory disorder.
- Look for signs of hidden haemorrhage, i.e. melaena.
- If the anaemia is the result of a poor diet, some food and health education may be recommended. It may also indicate poor social conditions where help needs to be offered.

ERYTHROCYTE SEDIMENTATION RATE

REFERENCE RANGE

Adult: less than 20 mm in 1 hour

Child: 2–10 mm in 1 hour

PROCEDURE

Venepuncture.

The specimen of blood should be sent to the laboratory immediately, as the erythrocytes will start to settle in the specimen tube, as it waits for collection.

CONTAINER

The specimen container used in this unit is:

PURPOSE

This measures the settlement rate of red blood cells as they fall to the bottom of a tube of unclotted blood, which has been left to stand for a predetermined length of time. It is only an indication of the presence of disease; it is not specific to any one disease process. It is the red blood cells and plasma proteins that influence the test results.

Increased sedimentation rates occur when:
- Infection or inflammatory disease is active. The number of plasma proteins will be increased, i.e. the immunoglobulins. This increased value of plasma proteins will cause the red cells to clump together as rouleau and these large red cell masses will fall to the bottom of the tube more rapidly.
- There is an increase in the red cell weight.

Decreased sedimentation rates occur when:
- The red blood cells are enlarged (macrocytic anaemia) and their rate of descent is slower.

Raised ESR may indicate:
– Inflammatory disease
– Collagen disease
– Auto-immune disease
– Chronic infection
– Neoplasms
– Post-trauma
– Pregnancy
– Ischaemia

Decreased ESR may indicate:
– Congestive cardiac failure
– Sickle cell anaemia
– Hypoproteinaemia
Drugs including:
– Steroids

DIFFERENTIAL WHITE CELL COUNT

REFERENCE RANGE

White blood cell (WBC) count.

Adult: $4–11 \times 10^9$/litre

Child: $4–12 \times 10^9$/litre

Neonate: $16–20 \times 10^9$/litre

PROCEDURE

Venepuncture.

CONTAINER

The specimen container used in this unit is:

PURPOSE

The differential white cell count quantifies each type of white cell present in the patient's blood. It expresses the presence of each type of leucocyte as a percentage of the total white cell blood count.

There are six different types of white blood cells or leucocytes:
- Lymphocytes   25–33%
- Monocytes   3–7%
- Neutrophils   57–63% ⎫
- Eosinophils   1–3% ⎬ Polymorphonuclear granulocytes
- Basophils   0.75% ⎭
- Plasma cells   Not usually included in the differential count.

Each type of leucocyte has its own characteristics and functions. This is reflected when changes in the white cell blood count become indicative of certain types of disease processes, e.g. eosinophil values will be raised if a parasitic infection is the reason for increased white blood cell activity in the body.

Lymphocytes are formed mainly in the lymphoid tissue, also in the bone marrow. They are needed for immunity against disease.

Monocytes are formed in the bone marrow.
They respond to tissue inflammation.

Granulocytes are formed and stored in the bone marrow.
They enter the circulatory system as a defence against inflammation, infection and toxic agents.

A *raised* white blood cell count usually indicates that the bone marrow has been stimulated as a defence mechanism. Stress and exercise will mobilise some of the sedentary white blood cells and cause an increase in circulating values.

A *lowered* white blood cell count indicates reduced white blood cell production from a depressed or diseased bone marrow.

ALTERED VALUES

RAISED WHITE BLOOD CELL (WBC) COUNT

Leucocytosis
- Stimulus to manufacture WBCs against infection, inflammation or immune response, e.g. bacterial infection
- Malignancy
- Dehydration
- Loss of plasma or fluids in which the circulating WBCs are diluted, e.g. burns
- Third trimester of pregnancy.

LOWERED WHITE CELL COUNT

Leucopenia
- Depressed bone marrow
- Acquired immune deficiency disease
- Agranulocytosis
- Auto-immune disease, e.g. systemic lupus erythematosus
- Reduced vitamin B12 or folic acid
- Overwhelming bacterial infection
- Viral infection.

OTHER ALTERED VALUES

Shift to the left
- The presence of immature granulocytes in the circulating blood associated with an acute stress on the bone marrow, e.g. bacterial infection, post-haemorrhage.

Shift to the right
- The nucleus of the neutrophils has an extra lobe. This can occur with Down's syndrome and pernicious anaemia.

Leucoerythroblastic anaemia
- The presence of myelocytes and normoblasts in the blood, usually with an accompanying anaemia. This indicates that the bone marrow is irritated, e.g. severe infections and myeloproliferative disorders.

Leukaemia
A raised number of abnormal white blood cells in the circulating blood. It is caused by a proliferation of leucocyte producing tissue, away from the normal sites of manufacture.

Agranulocytosis
The bone marrow stops production of granulocytes.

Pancytopenia
The number of circulating blood cells – white blood cells, red blood cells, platelets – is reduced. Either the bone marrow is failing or there is premature destruction of the cells.

REFERENCE RANGE

Adult: $1.5\text{--}4.0 \times 10^9$/litre

Child: $5.5\text{--}8.5 \times 10^9$/litre

Neonate: 5.5×10^9/litre

PROCEDURE

Venepuncture.

CONTAINER

The specimen container used in this unit is:

PURPOSE

To determine the number of lymphocytes in the circulating blood.

Lymphocytes give protection against invading organisms.

Lymphocytes are classified into two groups:

1. **T-lymphocytes**

T-lymphocytes are further divided according to their varying functions.
- The immunoregulatory helper (T_H) cells increase the activity of other types of lymphocytes.
- The cytotoxic (T_C) cells secrete enzymes into the invading organisms or malignant cells to destroy them.
- Suppressor (T_S) cells prevent the actions of T_C and T_H cells causing extensive damage.
- Delayed hypersensitive reaction (T_{DTH}) cells initiate a localised inflammatory response and activate macrophages.

2. **B-lymphocytes**

When stimulated by an antigen from an invading cell, the dormant B-cells proliferate and produce antibodies specifically designed to destroy the bacteria, virus, etc.

A rise in blood lymphocytes would normally mean that the immune response system has been stimulated.

NORMAL PHYSIOLOGY

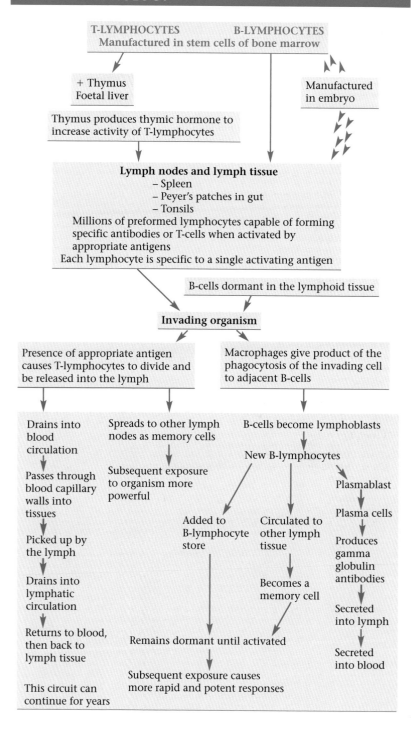

ALTERED VALUES

RAISED VALUES	LOWERED VALUES
Lymphocytosis	
Disease stimulus to increase lymphocyte production – Hyperthyroidism – Lymphosarcoma – Lymphocyte leukaemia	Diseases reducing lymphocyte production – Aplastic anaemia – Granulocytic and monocytic leukaemia
	Depressed lymphatic tissue – Post-radiation therapy
Immune response – Viral infections, e.g. whooping cough, infectious hepatitis – Bacterial infections – Chronic infection	Immune response – Leucopenia, reduced cells due to overwhelming infection
	Loss or destruction of lymphocytes – Systemic lupus erythematosus – Burns – Trauma
Effect of drugs, e.g. – Phenytoin	Effect of drugs, e.g. – Cortisone

REFERENCE RANGE

Adult: $0.04–0.4 \times 10^9$/litre

Child: 0.2×10^9/litre

Neonate: $0.2–0.9 \times 10^9$/litre

PROCEDURE

Venepuncture.

CONTAINER

The specimen container used in this unit is:

PURPOSE

To assess the eosinophil content of the blood.

Eosinophils are mainly concerned with allergic and parasitic conditions. Increased T-cell activity also stimulates production of eosinophils.

Eosinophils are granular cells. The granules contain materials that deactivate substances released during allergic reactions and parasitic infestations. Enzymes released by the eosinophil to destroy invading parasites may also damage healthy body tissues.

Eosinophils are also phagocytes. They have the ability to ingest material formed when antibodies and antigens meet.

NORMAL PHYSIOLOGY

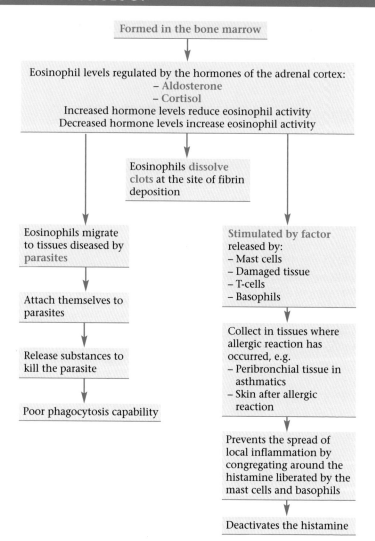

Formed in the bone marrow

Eosinophil levels regulated by the hormones of the adrenal cortex:
– Aldosterone
– Cortisol
Increased hormone levels reduce eosinophil activity
Decreased hormone levels increase eosinophil activity

Eosinophils dissolve clots at the site of fibrin deposition

Eosinophils migrate to tissues diseased by parasites

Attach themselves to parasites

Release substances to kill the parasite

Poor phagocytosis capability

Stimulated by factor released by:
– Mast cells
– Damaged tissue
– T-cells
– Basophils

Collect in tissues where allergic reaction has occurred, e.g.
– Peribronchial tissue in asthmatics
– Skin after allergic reaction

Prevents the spread of local inflammation by congregating around the histamine liberated by the mast cells and basophils

Deactivates the histamine

Lives for 12 hours in the blood and 20 hours in the tissues

ALTERED VALUES

RAISED VALUES

Eosinophilia

Excessive production
in bone marrow
– Eosinophilic leukaemia

Insufficient production of
adrenal cortical hormones
– Addison's disease

Neoplastic disorders
– Lymphoma
– Hodgkin's disease

Following radiation therapy

Allergic conditions
– Asthma
– Hay fever
– Urticaria
– Pulmonary eosinophilia

Parasitic conditions
– Malaria

Inflammatory conditions
– Dermatitis
– Rheumatoid arthritis

Eosinophilic fasciitis
A condition of the hands,
forearms and feet

Effects of drugs, including:
– Allopurinol

LOWERED VALUES

Eosinopenia

Decreased production in bone
marrow
– Aplastic anaemia

Overproduction of adrenal
cortical hormones
– Cushing's syndrome
– Increased ACTH production from the
  pituitary gland
– Stress

Hypersplenism

Congestive cardiac failure

Effects of drugs, including:
– Corticosteroid therapy

NEUTROPHILS

REFERENCE RANGE

Adult: $2.0–7.5 \times 10^9$/litre

Child: $1.5–7.0 \times 10^9$/litre

Neonate: 2.5×10^9/litre

PROCEDURE

Venepuncture.

CONTAINER

The specimen container used in this unit is:

PURPOSE

Neutrophils provide an important line of defence against invading organisms.

There are 4–5 times more neutrophils stored in the bone marrow than circulating in the blood.

When tissue becomes inflamed, it produces a hypersensitive reaction. This stimulates a chemical message to be sent to the bone marrow, to release more neutrophils into the blood.

Neutrophils are also manufactured, initiated by a substance produced by the macrophages, at the site of the inflamed tissue.

A pool of neutrophils lies along the epithelium of the blood vessels. They are mobilised to join the general circulation by the inflammatory response to the invading organism.

Neutrophils destroy the invading organisms by phagocytosis, an activity that also kills the short-lived neutrophil.

A *raised* neutrophil value is the normal body response to invasive agents.

A *lowered* neutrophil value occurs when neutrophils are not being manufactured in the bone marrow, a condition that makes the patient highly susceptible to infection.

NORMAL PHYSIOLOGY

Formed in bone marrow.

↓

Some released to circulate in the blood.
4–5 times more stored in the bone marrow.

↓

Invading organism inflames tissue.
Substances released in response to the damage.
Stimulates neutrophil release from the bone marrow.

↓

The neutrophils move to the inflamed area.
The neutrophils recognise the area of damage by:
– Substances released from the inflamed tissue attract the neutrophils.
– Capillary wall damage enhances the neutrophils' ability to stick to
  the blood vessel wall.
– Tissue damage increases the permeability of the capillary wall to
  allow neutrophils to pass through.

↓

Neutrophils can squeeze through capillary walls into the tissues. They
have an amoeboid action.

↓

In response to the breakdown products of bacterial toxins, neutrophils,
etc., macrophages produce a substance that stimulates the bone marrow
to manufacture more neutrophils.

↓

Neutrophils destroy small invading organisms by phagocytosis.
Neutrophils recognise the tissue to be destroyed by:
– The presence of a rough surface.
– The absence of a protective protein coat that surrounds normal tissue.
– As a foreign particle, immunoglobulin and complement attach
  themselves to the bacterial membrane. The neutrophils have receptors
  to recognise this as an indication to destroy the cell.

↓

The neutrophil is able to phagocytise 5–20 bacteria. When all of its
digestive enzymes and histamine granules have been used, the
neutrophil will die.

ALTERED VALUES

RAISED VALUES	LOWERED VALUES
Neutrophilia	**Neutropenia**
Bacterial infections, e.g. – Tonsillitis – Cellulitis	Reduced production due to disease of the bone marrow, e.g. – Acute lymphoblastic leukaemia – Aplastic anaemia – Agranulocytosis
Parasitic infection	
Inflammatory disorders, e.g. – Rheumatoid arthritis – Asthma	Acute viral infection
	At onset of infectious disease
Allergies	Destruction of the neutrophils in the circulating blood
Injections of foreign protein	Enlarged spleen – Lymphoma – Portal hypertension
Any tissue-damaging process, e.g. – Operative procedures – Myocardial infarction – Burns	
Stress – Emotional stress – Extreme fatigue	
Exercise Rapid blood flow mobilises the neutrophils on the capillary walls. This reverts to normal after one hour.	
Malignant tumours	
Diabetic acidosis	
Cushing's syndrome	Drugs, including: – Cytotoxic agents – Carbimazole – Sulphasalazine

REFERENCE RANGE

Adult: $0.01-0.1 \times 10^9$/litre

Child: 0.04×10^9/litre

Neonate: $0-0.6 \times 10^9$/litre

PROCEDURE

Venepuncture.

CONTAINER

The specimen container used in this unit is:

PURPOSE

To determine the basophil content of the blood.

Basophils are primarily concerned with allergic reactions. They also give some defence against worm parasites.

Inflammatory and hypersensitive conditions cause them to increase in number.

Basophils and mast cells are closely linked. Although basophils are circulating cells and mast cells remain within tissues, they share common origins and give similar responses to inflammatory and hypersensitive conditions.

NORMAL PHYSIOLOGY

Basophils are formed in the bone marrow.

They are similar to the mast cells that are found in tissues.

The **immunoglobulin IgE** has an affinity with the surface of basophils and mast cells. It becomes attached to the surface of basophils.

In response to contact with allergens, **IgE initiates an allergic response.**

When an allergen links to the IgE molecule, the basophils and mast cells rupture spilling out the granule content of the cell. This releases:
- Histamine
- Bradykinin
- Serotonin
- Heparin
- Lysosomal enzymes.

A local tissue and vascular tissue reaction results.

An allergic response is produced.

ALTERED VALUES

RAISED VALUES

Basophilia

Excessive production in
bone marrow
– Leukaemia

Hypothyroidism

Allergic reactions
– Food
– Drugs
– Environmental factors

Hodgkin's disease

Ulcerative colitis

Following splenectomy

Effect of drugs, including:
– Antithyroid drugs

LOWERED VALUES

Decreased production in
bone marrow
– Aplastic anaemia

Thyrotoxicosis
Overactive adrenal glands
– Cushing's disease
– Stress

Anaphylaxis

Acute infections

Pregnancy

Effect of drugs, including:
– Chemotherapy
– Corticosteroid therapy

MONOCYTES

REFERENCE RANGE

Adult: $0.2–0.8 \times 10^9$/litre

Child: $0.7–1.5 \times 10^9$/litre

Neonate: 1×10^9/litre

PROCEDURE

Venepuncture.

CONTAINER

The specimen container used in this unit is:

PURPOSE

To assess the number of monocytes that have been mobilised in response to inflamed or infected tissue.

There are few circulating monocytes, and these are usually in an immature state. As they reach their target tissue they pass through the capillary walls, enlarge, and mature into macrophages in order to fulfil their function.

Tissues contain their own characteristic macrophages, in permanent residence, e.g.:
- Kupffer cells in the liver
- Macrophages of the lung alveoli
- Microglial cells of the brain.

Inflammation attracts tissue macrophages; it also stimulates the bone marrow to manufacture monocytes, release them into the blood and increase the body's response to attack.

Macrophages have the ability to destroy large numbers of bacteria by phagocytosis.

They use the remnants of the ingested organisms to:
- Give information to lymphocytes for production of the correct antibody
- Stimulate the bone marrow to produce more immature monocytes.

Macrophages also:
- Cause the generalised systemic reaction to inflammation
- Destroy tumour cells.

A *raised* monocyte count suggests that an inflammatory condition is stimulating monocyte production.

Monocytes are formed in the bone marrow.

They have a short transit time in the blood as a small immature cell unable to fight infection.

They enter tissues through the blood capillary membranes, squeezing through pores and moving with an amoeboid action.

Other monocytes remain **stuck to the capillary wall**.

A monocyte enlarges by five times over 8–12 hours to become a macrophage, with the ability to phagocytise invading organisms.

Macrophages attach themselves to tissues and remain in place for years, unless called upon for specific purposes.

Inflamed tissue produces substances that:
- Attract macrophages to the inflamed area
- Stimulate the production and migration of more monocytes to the site.

These substances are:
- Bacterial toxins
- Products from inflamed tissue
- Reaction products of the complement complex
- Products of blood clotting.

The production of additional **T-cells** also activates macrophages.

A macrophage can destroy 100 bacteria by **phagocytosis** before it dies itself.

It is also able to engulf large particles, e.g.:
- Malarial parasites
- Necrotic tissue
- Dead neutrophils.

Macrophages also have the ability to destroy tumour cells.

The breakdown products resulting from the ingestion of invading organisms are passed from the macrophage to adjacent lymphocytes, so that they may develop the correct antibodies.

Macrophages aid healing by secreting substances that promote tissue repair.

ALTERED VALUES

RAISED VALUES	LOWERED VALUES

Monocytosis

Excessive production from diseased bone marrow – Leukaemia	Decreased production from diseased bone marrow – Aplastic anaemia
Acute bacterial infections	Chronic infections
Viral infections – Infectious mononucleosis	
Parasitic infections – Malaria	
Chronic inflammatory disorders – Subacute bacterial endocarditis – Rheumatoid arthritis – Ulcerative colitis	
Neoplastic disease – Tumours – Hodgkin's disease – Lymphoma	
	Effect of drugs, including: – Corticosteroid therapy

ASSOCIATED INVESTIGATIONS

		Related pages
Temperature	The presence of infection will cause a rise in temperature.	**4**
Differential white blood cell count	Changes in the differential white cell count can indicate the cause of the infection.	**44**
Haemoglobin Red blood cell count Platelets	Disease of the bone marrow will also affect the manufacture of white blood cells, red blood cells and platelets.	**38** **34** **63**
Blood film	The microscopic examination of the white blood cells.	
Swabs and cultures	Specimens to detect the source and type of infection. The organism's sensitivity to antibiotics will also be tested.	**293**
Assessment of symptoms	For example: ■ The presence of pain ■ Cough	
Bone marrow puncture	To investigate disease of the bone marrow, as the basis of a disordered white blood cell count.	**71**

WHITE CELL COUNT

CONSIDERATIONS FOR CARE

RAISED WHITE BLOOD CELL COUNT

The defence mechanisms of the body have been stimulated.

- The patient's conditions and symptoms should be assessed for the source of the reaction. Once the cause of the reaction is established, specific nursing care and treatments can be commenced.
- The patient's temperature will probably be raised. A regular temperature check will be needed. This is especially important for children under the age of five who risk febrile convulsions when their temperatures are raised.
- Barrier nursing precautions will need to be taken if the cause of the raised white cell count is, or suspected to be, infectious.
- Measures preventing cross-infection between patients will be needed.
- If an allergic reaction is the cause of the raised white cell count, and the causative allergen is unknown, a programme of sensitivity tests may be arranged.
- A raised white cell count may be caused by disordered cell production in the bone marrow. If this is suspected, the subsequent investigations are uncomfortable and stressful for the patient and their family.

LOWERED WHITE BLOOD CELL COUNT

A significantly reduced number of white blood cells will not provide the body with adequate defences. Protection against sources of acquired infection must be provided. The patient should be nursed in isolation, and maximum precautions must be taken to prevent contagion reaching them. Isolation may become distressing, especially if the patient has or is having treatment for serious illness.

It is important that:

- Patients are not allowed to feel neglected by their family, or the staff.
- Patients must still have regular visits to allow them to talk and voice their worries.
- The room must be kept fresh and comfortable, not allowing dirty crockery and other waste to collect.
- Sources of entertainment must be provided.

Care basic to health must be implemented:

- Good mouth care is essential.
- Care and comfort of the skin.
- Good nutrition in the form most acceptable to the patient.
- Comfortable bedding to help sleep and rest.

REFERENCE RANGE

Adult: $150–400 \times 10^9$/litre

Child: $200–500 \times 10^9$/litre

Neonate: $100–300 \times 10^9$/litre

PROCEDURE

Venepuncture.

If haemorrhagic disease is suspected avoid bruising by:
- Ensuring prompt removal of the tourniquet
- Minimal probing with the needle to locate the vein
- Applying prolonged pressure to the puncture site.

CONTAINER

The specimen container used in this unit is:

PURPOSE

To determine that the number of circulating platelets is within normal limits.

Platelets are disc-shaped, un-nucleated cells that circulate in the blood. They are also called 'thrombocytes'.

They have a sticky quality to their cell surface, allowing them to collect and adhere to each other and to the collagen exposed when a blood vessel wall is damaged. Once the platelet has become stuck into place, it releases other substances from granules in its cytoplasm, to continue the process of forming a platelet plug.

The platelet plug closes gaps and holes made in blood vessels when damage occurs.

The platelet plug forms the basis on which a blood clot can form.

A *lowered* platelet count would increase the risk of bleeding; stopping the bleeding may also be problematic.

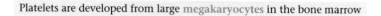

Platelets are developed from large megakaryocytes in the bone marrow

↓

Part of the cell elongates into a marrow blood sinusoid.
The tip of the extended part is nipped off – this is a platelet

↓

Taken into the blood circulation where it survives for 10 days

↓

When platelets come into contact with damaged tissue or a
blood vessel wall they aggregate around the injury. This is
facilitated by:
– Exposure of collagen in the vessel wall
– Factor XI
– Factor XII.

The platelets swell, become sticky and irregular in shape.

↓

The platelets begin to break down

↓

This breakdown, together with Factor VIII and Factor IX,
produces a platelet factor

↓

The following then occurs:
– A secreted activating substance causes nearby platelets to
  become sticky and adhere to the aggregation of platelets.
– Serotonin is released, causing local vasoconstriction.
– Platelet factor, Factors V and X, and the tissue injury initiates
  the formation of thromboplastin.

↓

The formation of the platelet plug, together with the
vasoconstriction, may stop the bleeding.

The thromboplastin produced will stimulate blood clotting.

ALTERED VALUES

RAISED VALUES

Thrombocytosis
Thrombocythaemia

Excessive platelet production
in the bone marrow
– Essential thrombocytosis
– Myelofibrosis
– Chronic myeloid leukaemia

Asphyxia

High altitudes

Chronic inflammatory disease
– Rheumatoid arthritis

Response to haemorrhage

Malignant disease
– Multiple myeloma
– Carcinoma

Following splenectomy

LOWERED VALUES

Thrombocytopenia

Decreased platelet production
in the bone marrow
Aplastic anaemia
Acute lymphocytic leukaemia
Myelofibrosis
Vitamin B12 or folate deficiency

Increased use while in circulation
Idiopathic thrombocytopenia purpura
Disseminated intravascular coagulation

Irradiation

Prior to menstruation

Excessive destruction by the spleen
Liver disease

Effect of drugs, including:

– Indometacin
– Mefenamic acid
– Cimetidine
– Sulfasalazine

PROTHROMBIN

REFERENCE RANGE

Prothrombin time – Adult: 12–16 s
                 Child: 11–14 s
                 Neonate: 12–18 s

International normalised ratio (INR) 1

$$INR = \frac{\text{Patient's prothrombin time in seconds}}{\text{Mean normal prothrombin time in seconds}}$$

PROCEDURE

Venepuncture.

The specimen must be sent promptly for processing.

The specimen must not be refrigerated.

If poor blood clotting ability is suspected, apply firm, prolonged pressure to the skin puncture to prevent bruising.

Check the site until certain that no further bleeding will occur.

CONTAINER

The specimen container used in this unit is:

PURPOSE

Prothrombin time is measured to assess the clotting ability of the patient's blood. Prothrombin is Factor II in the cascade mechanism of blood coagulation.

Prothrombin is a plasma protein. It is inactive until tissue damage begins a reaction that converts prothrombin to its active form, **thrombin**. The measurement of prothrombin time assesses the competence of the component parts in this preliminary stage of blood clotting.

Patients needing anticoagulant therapy have prothrombin time measured regularly to monitor their blood clotting times and as an assessment of correct drug dosage.

A *raised* prothrombin time would indicate a shorter blood clotting time.

A *lowered* prothrombin time would indicate a longer time is taken for the blood to clot.

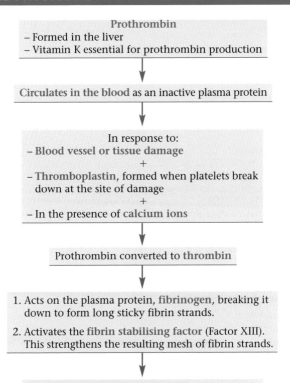

Prothrombin
- Formed in the liver
- Vitamin K essential for prothrombin production

↓

Circulates in the blood as an inactive plasma protein

↓

In response to:
- Blood vessel or tissue damage
  +
- Thromboplastin, formed when platelets break down at the site of damage
  +
- In the presence of calcium ions

↓

Prothrombin converted to thrombin

↓

1. Acts on the plasma protein, fibrinogen, breaking it down to form long sticky fibrin strands.

2. Activates the fibrin stabilising factor (Factor XIII). This strengthens the resulting mesh of fibrin strands.

↓

The sticky mesh of fibrin threads:
- Adhere to the edges of the damaged tissue
- Trap blood cells, platelets and plasma proteins.

The clot is formed.

PROTHROMBIN TIME

INCREASED	DECREASED
Lowered prothrombin value	Raised prothrombin value
Liver disease – Hepatitis – Cirrhosis	Arterial occlusion
	Deep vein thrombosis
Vitamin K deficiency – Neonates lack intestinal flora needed for the synthesis of vitamin K – Vitamin K is absorbed in the blood with digested fats; poor fat absorption = poor vitamin K absorption – Biliary obstruction – Obstructive jaundice – Malabsorption	Myocardial infarction
	Pulmonary embolus
Deficiency of other factors relevant to the action of prothrombin, during clot formation – Afibrinogenaemia – Factor deficiency – Low platelet count	
Snake bite	
Effect of drugs, including: – Anticoagulant therapy – Heparin – Aspirin	Effect of drugs, including: – Oral contraceptives

PLATELETS AND PROTHROMBIN

ASSOCIATED INVESTIGATIONS

		Related pages
Blood film	The microscopic examination of the platelets.	
Bleeding time	The careful recording of the time the blood takes to clot at a point of injury (3–10 min).	
Activated partial thromboplastin time	Stimulates and assesses the capability of the blood clotting mechanism.	
Thrombin time		
Bone marrow puncture	To examine the maturation of platelets.	**71**

The presence of clotting factors		
	Factor I	Fibrinogen
	Factor II	Prothrombin
	Factor III	Tissue thromboplastin
	Factor IV	Calcium ions
	Factor V	Labile factor
	Factor VI	None
	Factor VII	Stable factor
	Factor VIII	Antihaemophilic factor
	Factor IX	Christmas factor
	Factor X	Stuart-Prower factor
	Factor XI	Plasma thromboplastin antecedent
	Factor XII	Hageman factor
	Factor XIII	Fibrin stabilising factor.

Marks on skin Evidence of internal bleeding	Haemorrhage, bruising, petechiae, purpura.	

CONSIDERATIONS FOR CARE

INCREASED RISK OF BLEEDING

– **Decreased number or function of platelets**
– **Increased prothrombin time**

The carer must constantly be aware of the patient's tendency to bleed during nursing and medical intervention. Skin punctures and procedures where abrasions may occur to the mucous membranes, i.e. passing a nasogastric tube, may be hazardous.

Teeth cleaning, shaving and other everyday activities will need care.

Risk of accidents must be minimised. The environment around the patient should be modified according to the patient's mobility and abilities, to ensure their safety.

Constant observation to detect signs of bleeding will be needed.

Specimens of stool and urine must be routinely tested for blood, to detect covert bleeding.

If haemorrhage is detected, immediate action is necessary to stop the flow and replace circulatory volume, if required.

Regular monitoring of pulse, respirations and blood pressure will be needed.

If haemorrhage has occurred, remove all signs of blood as quickly as possible to reduce patient anxiety. Old blood will also be a source of infection. Give appropriate personal hygiene care to clear the skin or mouth of blood.

Monitoring, following surgery or other invasive procedures, must be vigilant.

Blood or blood products may be given intravenously to the patient to improve blood clotting ability. Stop the infusion immediately if the patient has an adverse reaction, detected by a rise in temperature or the appearance of a skin rash.

INCREASED RISK OF BLOOD CLOTTING

– **Increased number of platelets**
– **Decreased prothrombin time**

The underlying condition causing the increased number of platelets, or decreasing the prothrombin time, must be treated.

Planned patient care must decrease the risk of the formation of blood clots. Maximum mobilisation to the patient's own limits will be needed to promote the flow of blood through blood vessels.

If it is difficult for the patient to leave his or her bed or chair, a programme of passive movements and exercises should be devised with support to encourage the regular use of the exercises. Physiotherapy will be beneficial.

Tight bands around the patient's limbs must be avoided.

Red bone marrow is the site of production and maturation of red blood cells, white blood cells and platelets.

A tissue sample is taken from the bone marrow to view these processes:
- To ensure that the cells are produced in their correct numbers
- To ensure that the cells follow correct maturation processes before entering the blood.

PROCEDURE

The collection of bone marrow must follow local policy and procedures.

The bone marrow is collected from the sternum or the iliac crest. It is an uncomfortable and worrying procedure for the patient. Full supportive care must be available to the patient during the procedure in addition to the medical staff required to remove the bone marrow.

A full explanation of the procedure should be given to the patient before starting. Prior warning of the expected unpleasant sensations associated with the practice must be explained, together with the assurance that measures will be taken to help the patient tolerate the process.

Full aseptic technique must be used.

The specimen must be sent to the laboratory immediately.

The puncture site on the skin must be sealed and protected from infection.

PURPOSE

To scrutinise the maturation processes of the red blood cells, white blood cells and platelets.

The blood cells have a common origin, from the stem cells found in the bone marrow. The red bone marrow is found in the ends of the long bones, in the flat bones and in the ribs.

Although the stem cells provide the common starting point for cell maturation, the various types of cells rely on different stimuli to initiate their production. Conditions that interfere with blood cell production are described within this book, in the sections specific to each type of cell.

Bone marrow transplantation, using the patient's own marrow or marrow of the same tissue type, can be remedial in malignant disease.

If the transplant is successful, it can provide resistance to the remaining malignant cells. It also provides healthier marrow on which therapeutic agents can work.

TOTAL PROTEIN

REFERENCE RANGE

Adult: 62–80 g/l

Child: 52–78 g/l

Neonate: 44–63 g/l

PROCEDURE

Venepuncture.

CONTAINER

The specimen container used in this unit is:

PURPOSE

To measure the blood plasma protein value.

This information is limited as a reference point, as there are three main types of plasma protein present in the blood:
- Albumin
- Globulins
- Fibrinogen.

The total protein measurement will be distorted if any of the protein types are recording abnormal values.

Separate assessment of each of these proteins would be needed to clarify an abnormal total protein result.

The different types of plasma protein provide a wide variety of functions.

Their main uses are:
- For materials that bind themselves to proteins as a medium for transport in the blood circulation, e.g. hormones, vitamins, enzymes.
- They provide replacement proteins when tissues need building or repair.
- They provide an osmotic pull; this attracts water from the tissues and channels it back into the capillaries. This ensures a correct volume of circulating water is maintained.
- They are buffers, part of the mechanism that maintains body pH at 7.4.
- Globulins provide immunity.
- Fibrinogen is part of the blood clotting system.

A *raised* total protein indicates that one or more of the protein constituents in the plasma is at a higher than normal value.

A *lowered* total protein indicates that one or more of the protein constituents in the blood is at a lower than normal value.

The physical effects of these changes will largely depend on the protein that is at the incorrect value. Results will be affected by recent administration of protein products, i.e. blood transfusions and vaccinations.

NORMAL PHYSIOLOGY

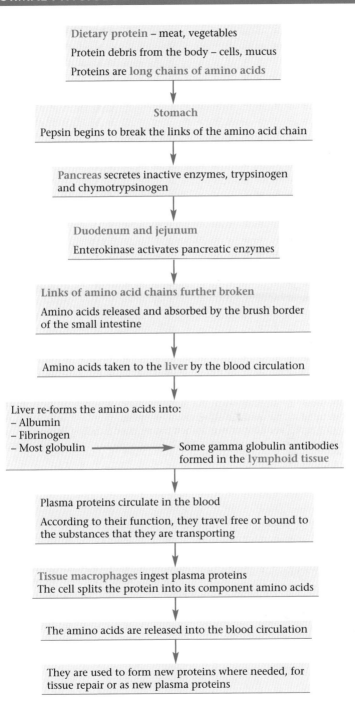

Dietary protein – meat, vegetables

Protein debris from the body – cells, mucus

Proteins are long chains of amino acids

Stomach

Pepsin begins to break the links of the amino acid chain

Pancreas secretes inactive enzymes, trypsinogen and chymotrypsinogen

Duodenum and jejunum

Enterokinase activates pancreatic enzymes

Links of amino acid chains further broken

Amino acids released and absorbed by the brush border of the small intestine

Amino acids taken to the liver by the blood circulation

Liver re-forms the amino acids into:
– Albumin
– Fibrinogen
– Most globulin ⟶ Some gamma globulin antibodies formed in the lymphoid tissue

Plasma proteins circulate in the blood

According to their function, they travel free or bound to the substances that they are transporting

Tissue macrophages ingest plasma proteins
The cell splits the protein into its component amino acids

The amino acids are released into the blood circulation

They are used to form new proteins where needed, for tissue repair or as new plasma proteins

ALTERED VALUES

RAISED VALUES	LOWERED VALUES
Haemoconcentration – Dehydration – Vomiting – Diarrhoea	Inadequate dietary protein – Malnutrition – Protein deprivation – Malabsorption
	Liver disease
Multiple myeloma	Loss of proteins – Haemorrhage – Severe burns
Chronic infection	
Chronic inflammatory disease	
	Protein loss through gastrointestinal tract – Crohn's disease – Ulcerative colitis
	Protein loss through renal system – Chronic glomerulonephritis – Nephrotic syndrome – Proteinuria
Effect of drugs, including: – Steroids	Effect of drugs, including: – Oral contraceptives

REFERENCE RANGE

Adult: 34–48 g/l

Child: 35–50 g/l

Neonate: 33–45 g/l

PROCEDURE

Venepuncture.

CONTAINER

The container used in this unit is:

PURPOSE

To measure the plasma protein, albumin, circulating in the blood.

Albumin is one of the three main types of plasma protein.

Of these three, albumin is the plasma protein that is present in the greatest amount.

It is manufactured by the liver. As the half life of albumin is relatively long (20–26 days), the physical effects of a reduced albumin level are delayed.

The presence of albumin in the capillaries provides the osmotic pull that attracts and holds water in the blood vessels. This counteracts the forces exerted by the intravascular blood pressure and the tissues surrounding the capillary, forcing the water to leave blood vessels and move into the tissues.

A decreased albumin content will upset this balance and too much water will move into the tissues. Oedema will result.

Albumin has binding sites to transport other substances circulating in the blood safely, e.g. hormones, enzymes and bilirubin.

Albumin levels are a good indicator of hepatic function. Sequential decreasing albumin values infer that the liver is gradually failing in its function.

ALTERED VALUES

RAISED VALUES	LOWERED VALUES
Haemoconcentration – Dehydration – Vomiting – Diarrhoea – Burns	Inadequate dietary protein – Malnutrition – Malabsorption
Neoplasms – Multiple myeloma – Carcinomatosis	Neoplasms – Lymphoma – Leukaemia
Inflammatory conditions – Rheumatoid arthritis – Polyarteritis	Decreased production – Chronic liver disease
Stress	Oedematous conditions – Ascites – Congestive cardiac failure
	Loss of albumin – Through gastrointestinal tract (ulcerative colitis) – Through the renal tract (nephrotic syndrome) – Haemorrhage
Effect of drugs, including: – Cytotoxic drugs	

REFERENCE RANGE

Adult: 15–35 g/l

Child: 17–28 g/l

Neonate: 9–22 g/l

The measurement of globulin can be further reduced by the itemising of the various types of protein that are classified as globulins.

PROCEDURE

Venepuncture.

CONTAINER

The specimen container used in this unit is:

PURPOSE

To measure the globulin components of the blood.

They are larger cells than albumin.

They are produced by the liver and lymphoid tissue.

Globulin takes many different forms.

Glycoproteins or alpha-1 and alpha-2 globulins

These molecules combine carbohydrates and protein.

The carbohydrate element of this globulin projects from the cell surface. This provides binding sites on which substances can attach themselves for transportation in the blood (transport proteins).

Lipoproteins or beta globulins

These molecules combine lipids and proteins.

It is their function to provide transport for circulating lipids.

These blood values are altered by a high fat diet.

Immunoglobulins or gamma globulins

These are produced in the lymphoid tissue as a body defence.

Invading organisms produce antigens that stimulate the production of the immunoglobulins or antibodies.

They take the form of IgMs, IgEs, IgAs, IgGs, and IgDs.

Each group of antibodies has a different purpose when protecting the body against infections, toxins and allergies.

These values are altered by recent immunisations and transfusions.

ALTERED VALUES

RAISED VALUES	LOWERED VALUES
Hyperglobulinaemia	**Hypoglobulinaemia**
Alpha-1 globulins	Alpha-1 globulins
Haemoconcentration	Decreased dietary intake of protein
– dehydration	Malabsorption
Hypoproteinaemia	Viral hepatitis
– Liver disease	
	Loss of protein through disease
Metastatic disease	– Nephrotic syndrome
Diabetes mellitus	– Ulcerative colitis
Acute inflammation	
– Glomerulonephritis	
Alpha-2 globulins	Alpha-2 globulins
Acute infection or	Reduced dietary intake of protein
inflammation	Malabsorption
Lack of adrenal hormones	Viral hepatitis
Leukaemia	Loss of protein through disease
	– Nephrotic syndrome
	– Ulcerative colitis
Beta globulins	Beta globulins
Haemoconcentration	Reduced dietary intake of proteins
– Dehydration	Malabsorption
Liver disease	– Steatorrhoea
– Cirrhosis	Loss of protein through disease
Cushing's disease	– Nephrotic syndrome
Obstructive jaundice	– Ulcerative colitis
Diabetes mellitus	Autoimmune disease
	– Subacute lupus erythematosus
Gamma globulins	Gamma globulins
Haemoconcentration	Reduced dietary intake of proteins
– Dehydration	Malabsorption
Liver disease	Asthma
Chronic infection and	Allergies
inflammation	Cushing's disease
Chronic lymphatic leukaemia	Loss of protein through disease
Cystic fibrosis	– Nephrotic syndrome
Neoplasms and metastases	– Ulcerative colitis

PLASMA PROTEINS

ASSOCIATED INVESTIGATIONS

		Related pages
Tests of liver function: ■ Serum bilirubin ■ Liver transaminases ■ Prothrombin time	Tests the ability of the liver to manufacture plasma proteins.	211
Plasma protein electrophoresis	Identifies the types of proteins present in specimen.	
Tests for proteinuria: ■ Reagent stick ■ 24-hour collection of urine	Identifies abnormal loss of protein through the renal system.	72
Blood urea	Quantifies the breakdown of proteins by the liver, for excretion.	121
Test of protein malabsorption: ■ 3-day stool collection	Identifies a problem with the absorption of dietary protein.	
Differential white cell count	Identifies the presence of inflammation or infection; this will alter globulin levels.	44
Examination of oedematous tissue	■ The sites of oedematous tissue on the body ■ The ability to leave a dent or 'pit' the oedema by pressing it with a finger.	44
Laboratory examination of ascites fluid	Microscopic investigation of cells: ■ Cell types present ■ Quantities of cells present ■ Staining and culture for bacteria.	283

CONSIDERATIONS FOR CARE

RAISED PLASMA PROTEIN VALUES

A lack of circulating water to dilute the number of plasma proteins will artificially raise the grams of protein per litre of blood. The patient must therefore be further examined for signs of dehydration.

The cause of a true rise in plasma proteins may be infectious, inflammatory or neoplastic in nature and will require immediate treatment.

An increase in circulating glucocorticoids will initiate increased protein metabolism. Steroid therapy or hypersecretion of glucocorticoids from the adrenal cortex will take protein from body tissue and use it for gluconeogenesis. The rise in circulating proteins will mask the reduced nature of the muscle and tissue proteins. An increase in the protein content of the diet will be needed to supplement this loss.

DECREASED PLASMA PROTEIN VALUES

If the patient's diet is found to be lacking in sufficient protein, the reasons and remedy should be sought. For changes in diet to be adopted, the patient must understand and approve the changes that are suggested.

Liver and kidney disease may cause a loss of protein. Replacement protein given orally or intravenously can be given to bring plasma and tissue protein back to normal values.

Reduced values of plasma proteins, especially albumin, cause fluid retention in the tissues. This fluid will drain to collect in definite areas of the body causing, for example, swollen oedematous ankles and abdominal ascites.

When a patient shows signs of oedema, an accurate fluid intake and output chart must be maintained. Even though fluid is remaining in the tissues, there must also be adequate circulatory fluid to maintain a normal blood volume.

Sufficient fluid must continue to circulate through the kidneys, to clear waste products and attempt to maintain pH, electrolyte and fluid balance.

The patient may be prescribed diuretic therapy and its effectiveness must be assessed by:
- Daily weight measurement – to detect any rapid gain or loss of weight associated with the retention or loss of fluid
- Daily girth measurement – using the same marked diameter will indicate a resolution or resumption of ascites.

The high water and the low protein content of body tissues will make them very susceptible to damage. Skin and pressure area care become essential.

TYPES

Blood groups:

	A Rh +ve	A Rh −ve
	B Rh +ve	B Rh −ve
	AB Rh +ve	AB Rh −ve
	O Rh +ve	O Rh −ve

PROCEDURE

Venepuncture.

CONTAINER

The specimen container used in this unit is:

PURPOSE

To identify the blood group of an individual, prior to being a prospective recipient of blood or blood donor.

Before donated blood is transfused into a recipient, compatibility must be determined.

Identification of blood groups depends on the presence, or absence, of:
- **Agglutinins** in the plasma
- **Agglutinogens** on the red blood cells.

A mismatched transfusion will cause incompatible agglutinins and agglutinogens to meet, initiating the clumping together of red blood cells.

The effects of this will be:
- The plugging of small blood vessels with clumped cells
- Haemolysis, or breakdown, of the clumped red blood cells, which will release haemoglobin into the circulation. This will block renal tubules.

Circulatory shock and jaundice will follow.

The presence of plasma agglutinins varies with age:
- Birth–2 months – virtually none
- 2–8 months – agglutinin production begins
- 8–10 years – maximum levels.

There is then a gradual decline with age until levels are very low in old age.

NORMAL PHYSIOLOGY

The typing of blood depends on the presence (or absence) of factors that, if allowed to meet, will cause the red blood cells to agglutinate or clump together.

These factors are:

Agglutinogens found on the red blood cell
Agglutinins found in the plasma.

If an agglutinin meets its agglutinogen, the red cells will clump together.

BLOOD GROUP	AGGLUTINOGEN (red blood cell)	AGGLUTININ (plasma)
A	A	Anti-B
B	B	Anti-A
AB	A and B	None
O	None	Anti-A and Anti-B

RHESUS FACTOR

A rhesus-negative (Rh −ve) person will make their own rhesus agglutinogen (anti-D), if rhesus-positive (Rh +ve) blood enters their blood circulation.

The first transfusion has no effect. The second and subsequent transfusion will cause red cell agglutination.

An example of this reaction occurs when a Rh +ve baby is born to a Rh −ve mother. Leakage of the baby's blood into the maternal circulation will cause the mother to develop rhesus agglutinogen (anti-D), an antibody that will react against rhesus (D) +ve blood.

The first baby will be unaffected.

If the second or subsequent baby is Rh −ve, no reaction will occur.
If this baby is Rh +ve, the maternal agglutinogen (anti-D) will cause the destruction of the baby's red blood cells.

This situation is now preventable.

Rhesus −ve mothers can be given an injection of anti-D immunoglobulin. This destroys any D-antigen that has entered the maternal circulation from a previous Rh +ve baby. The maternal blood is then free from the antibody that would harm her next baby.

ASSOCIATED INVESTIGATIONS

		Related pages
Cross-matching	Laboratory tests to confirm the compatibility of the blood for transfusion and the recipient's blood.	**81**
Haemoglobin Full blood count	Donated blood must conform to normal expected component values. Blood or blood products may be transfused when the recipient has a reduced haemoglobin or deficient blood cell counts.	**38**
Serum bilirubin	A product formed when red cells break down. This is a significant test when deciding on the treatment of neonatal jaundice.	**211**
Coombs' test	Blood is taken from the umbilical cord, when a baby is born to a mother with Rh −ve blood. The test will show the presence of antibodies attached to the red blood cells in the foetal circulation.	
Kleihauer test	Rh −ve maternal blood is tested post-delivery for the presence of Rh +ve foetal cells.	

CONSIDERATIONS FOR CARE

Transfusions of blood and blood products must be carefully monitored. Infusions of whole blood, blood cells, proteins or plasma carry the risk of initiating a poor reaction by the patient.

PRIOR TO INFUSION

As far as it is possible, the patient should be fully prepared for the infusion.

Attention must be given to their comfort as they will be restricted in movement for the duration of the infusion.

Full explanation of procedures must be given to the patient at all points of the procedure.

The following should be checked:
- The venous cannula is patent
- The cannula is properly placed in the lumen of the vein
- The patient's arm is kept still, in a good position. This reduces the risk of displacing the tip of the cannula, from the vein into surrounding tissue. Movement may also occlude the flow of blood through the cannula.

The blood or blood product must be in a good condition when it is transfused. Cells disintegrate when they are kept in the wrong environment.

Blood must be stored correctly prior to use, and must be used without delay when it arrives in the department for transfusion.

The checks that ensure the correct blood has been sent for the patient must be made according to local policy and practice.

Gloves should be worn by all staff handling the packs of blood.

DURING THE INFUSION

A prescribed infusion rate must be set and the rate of flow adjusted accordingly.

Regular observations of the patient's temperature, pulse and respirations must be made.

An initial blood pressure recording may be useful, from which comparisons may be made if the patient's condition deteriorates during transfusion. A rise in temperature and pulse may indicate an incompatibility between the patient's own blood and the infused blood. Loin pain, restlessness, a skin rash and haematuria may also become apparent.

A fluid input and output chart must be maintained. This will record the exact amount of infusion received by the patient. It will also demonstrate the adequacy of the patient's kidneys to deal with the additional circulating fluid.

If the kidneys are unable to excrete sufficient surplus water, the volume of fluid in the patient's circulation will rise. If the infusion continues, circulatory volume will become excessive, initiating a rise in the respiratory and pulse rate.

For the safety of all staff, dispose of all blood products and equipment according to hospital policy.

BLOOD GLUCOSE

REFERENCE RANGE

Adult: 4.5–5.6 mmol/l

Child: 3.4–5.6 mmol/l

Neonate: 2.6–5.0 mmol/l

PROCEDURE

Venepuncture.

Capillary blood for glucometer.

CONTAINER

The specimen container used in this unit is:

PURPOSE

The accurate measurement of blood glucose.

Dietary carbohydrates are reduced to glucose by digestion, for absorption and circulation in the blood.

Glucose and oxygen together provide energy for cells to function. The end product of this reaction is carbon dioxide and water.

Insulin mediates the passage of glucose across cell walls. It is within the mitochondria of the cell that glucose is used for energy production. Insulin also puts surplus glucose into store, in the form of glycogen. Glucagon, from the pancreas, brings glucose out of storage when the available circulating glucose is becoming low.

Adrenaline and cortisone are among the hormones that work in opposition to insulin in the regulation of blood glucose levels. They have the power to increase the release of glycogen, and convert it back to glucose.

The use of glucose by brain cells is not mediated by insulin. Glucose diffuses directly through the brain cell walls. This makes the brain very vulnerable to changes in blood glucose levels. When extreme blood glucose limits are reached, whether raised or lowered, normal brain function is interrupted, and unconsciousness can follow.

Pregnancy-induced hyperglycaemia or gestational diabetes is a temporary condition that is resolved with the birth of the baby.

Blood glucose values rise immediately after a meal, then fall to a fasting level 2 hours later.

MEASUREMENT USING A HAND-HELD GLUCOMETER

Hand-held glucometers are a convenient method of determining glucose values. Collecting blood for testing will require a capillary stab which can give discomfort, especially when repeated testing is necessary.

They are used:
- For repeated monitoring when attempting to stabilise blood glucose
- For routine monitoring of controlled diabetes mellitus
- For detection of hypoglycaemia and hyperglycaemia in the newborn
- To eliminate diabetes mellitus as the cause of presenting symptoms, i.e. unconsciousness.

The procedure must:
- Follow locally agreed policies and practices
- Be used in accordance with instructions issued by the manufacturer of the glucometer.

The following points will also apply to a baby's heel when glucometers are used to monitor the blood glucose value of a newborn.
- The finger should be clean, before the skin is pricked.
- Warm the finger to dilate the blood vessels to allow the drop of blood to flow more freely from the finger tip.
- The blood should not be massaged from the wound. The damage to the tissues with subsequent seepage of tissue fluid will give a false result.
- Avoid areas that show evidence of previous test stabs. The finger tips can become very sore.
- There must be sufficient blood for the glucometer to work accurately.
- Correct timekeeping during the test is essential for accuracy.
- Make sure that the wound has stopped bleeding before leaving the patient.
- Make use of interventions that make the procedure less painful.
- Children who are newly diagnosed diabetics, and their parents, will need special encouragement to cope with this procedure.

NORMAL PHYSIOLOGY

Dietary intake of carbohydrate

↓

Starch and sugars reduced to glucose by the action of digestive enzymes in the small intestine

↓

Glucose is absorbed into the blood circulation by the small intestine

↓

Insulin is released from the islet cells of the pancreas.
The main stimulators of insulin release are:
– Food in the stomach
– A raised blood glucose level
Insulin:
– Enhances the diffusion of glucose into cells
– Ensures the use of glucose as the energy source for cell metabolism
– Maintains a normal blood glucose level by storing circulating glucose that is not immediately required

↓

Circulating blood glucose diffuses through cell walls

↓

Glucose and oxygen follow a pathway of reactions in the cells.
This pathway provides energy for the metabolic activities needed for life.
Carbon dioxide and water are waste products of this process.

↓

Excess glucose stored as

Lipogenesis

↓

Converted to fat and put into store

Liver glycogen

Easily reconverted to glucose when the blood glucose level needs to be raised

↓

Reconverted by the action of glucagon released from the pancreas:
– In the absence of insulin
– In times of stress or prolonged exercise

Muscle glycogen

Can not be reconverted to maintain blood glucose levels

↓

It can only be used as a source of energy when the muscle exercises

ALTERED VALUES

RAISED VALUES	LOWERED VALUES
Hyperglycaemia	**Hypoglycaemia**
Decreased insulin production – Diabetes mellitus – Pancreatic insufficiency	Excess production of insulin – Pancreatic islet cell tumour
	Overdose of administered insulin
Endocrine disorders – Hyperthyroidism – Hyperadrenalism – Hyperpituitarism	Endocrine disorders – Addison's disease – Hypopituitarism – Hypothyroidism

Stress, causing release of adrenaline
– Anaesthesia
– Convulsions
– Shock
– Sudden illness, i.e.
  myocardial infarction,
  cerebrovascular accident
– Trauma
	Exercise

	Reduced dietary glucose – Malnutrition – Vomiting
	Prolonged fever
	Hypothermia
Pregnancy	Newborn baby of diabetic mother
Eclampsia	
Hypertension	Liver disease – Cirrhosis – Alcoholism
Chronic infection	
Meningitis	
Obesity	
Effect of drugs, including: – Cimetidine – Corticosteroids – Imipramine – Indometacin	Effects of drugs, including: – Insulin

ASSOCIATED INVESTIGATIONS

Related pages

Glycosylated haemoglobin assay (HbA1c)	Glucose combines with a particular type of haemoglobin in the red blood cell. This attachment of glucose is not reversible and is not altered in the short term by diet and medication. The life of a red blood cell is 120 days and the examined blood will give an indication of the blood glucose values during that previous length of time. A raised glycosylated haemoglobin value will indicate prolonged, poorly controlled diabetes mellitus. Anaemia and pregnancy will interfere with the accuracy of the test.	
Urine testing for glucose	Glucose is not normally present in the urine. When the blood glucose level is high, glucose is excreted through the kidneys.	85
Urine testing for ketones	Ketones are not normally present in the urine. When insulin is not available to use glucose for cell metabolism, fats provide the source of energy. The by-product of this process are ketones. They are excreted through the urine.	197
Blood pH	The presence of ketones in the blood will lower the blood pH – a state of acidosis.	150
Signs of infection	Raised temperature, inflammation. Candidiasis.	
Signs of dehydration	Glucose acts as an osmotic diuretic as it is excreted through the kidneys.	
Respirations	The presence of ketones in the blood lowers the body pH. The lungs try to correct this condition by ridding the body of carbon dioxide. Respirations will increase in rate and depth. The distinctive smell of ketones will be on the breath.	129
Glucose tolerance test	Following the intake of a measured dose of glucose, blood samples are taken over a regulated period of time. This will show abnormalities in the use of glucose by the body.	
Level of consciousness	Hyperglycaemia and hypoglycaemia will cause the brain cells to lose their function.	262
Fluid input and output chart	Glucose in the urine will act as an osmotic diuretic and increase urinary output. This will cause a thirst and polydipsia.	

CONSIDERATIONS FOR CARE

RAISED BLOOD GLUCOSE (HYPERGLYCAEMIA)

Diminished insulin production will have caused the blood glucose to rise. The patient may have felt various effects of this, e.g. polyuria, polydipsia, recurring infection and tiredness. If blood glucose rises to an excessive value, the patient will become unrousable from sleep. Immediate steps must be taken to reduce the blood glucose to avoid permanent neurological damage.

The patient will need help to understand the nature of diabetes mellitus. They will need to appreciate the balance between their diet, their insulin prescription and the amount of exercise they take.

This understanding must extend to:
- Safely administering a correct dose of insulin at the right time
- Measuring and recording their own blood glucose at regular intervals, and recognising normal parameters
- Knowing the type and quantities of food that make up a safe diet.

The patient should experience a hypoglycaemic episode and provide a remedy for it.

The patient should be comfortable with self-monitoring of blood glucose values using hand-held glucometers. Urine testing for glucose can be used although the first urine specimen of the morning will not be an accurate measurement of glucose levels.

LOW BLOOD GLUCOSE (HYPOGLYCAEMIA)

When blood glucose is found to be under normal set limits, glucose needs to be given promptly.

Brain cells can not operate without glucose and, if this is not available, the brain will cease to function. Sweating, headache and disorientation may be initial signs of hypoglycaemia. Unconsciousness and death will follow if left untreated.

The method of administering the glucose will depend on the condition of the patient. It can be given intravenously, nasogastrically or orally.

A record must be kept of the amount of glucose given and the time it took for the patient to recover.

THYROXINE (T4) AND TRI-IODOTHYRONINE (T3)

REFERENCE RANGE

Adult: Total serum thyroxine: 60–160 nmol/l
          Tri-iodothyronine: 1.2–3.1 nmol/l

Child: Total serum thyroxine: 83–172 nmol/l
          Tri-iodothyronine: 1.45–3.71 nmol/l

Neonate: Total serum thyroxine: 90–200 nmol/l
          Tri-iodothyronine: 0.4–3.33 nmol/l

PROCEDURE

Venepuncture.

CONTAINER

The specimen container used in this unit is:

PURPOSE

The measurements of thyroxine and tri-iodothyronine are part of a sequence of assessments that test the function of the **thyroid gland.**

It is the release and use of thyroxine and tri-iodothyronine from the thyroid gland that regulate the pace of cellular activities. A general increase, or decrease, of reaction speed at cell level will be apparent in the performance of the whole body.

Tri-iodothyronine is the hormone that determines the metabolic activity of cells. Thyroxine is thought to be a prohormone that needs to be converted to tri-iodothyronine before it can be used.

Tri-iodothyronine attaches to the appropriate receptor sites on the cells. These attachments regulate the speed at which glucose and lipids are used to provide energy for cellular activities.

Cell metabolism is basic to every function of life, including nutrition, respiration, growth and reproduction. Under normal circumstances, tri-iodothyronine will stimulate these processes at an appropriate rate. Diseases that affect the secretion or carriage of thyroid hormones will alter the rate of cell metabolism.

An *increase* in the amount of circulating thyroid hormones will increase the metabolic rate. An increase in speed of nearly all physical and mental body functions will become apparent.

A *decrease* in the amount of circulating thyroid hormones will slow the pace of mental and physical functions.

The **sympathetic nervous system** also has an influence on the speed of intracellular processes.

NORMAL PHYSIOLOGY

Hypothalamus
When stimulated secretes:
– Thyrotrophin releasing hormone
– Somatostatin, an inhibitor of thyroid stimulating hormone

Anterior pituitary gland
Releases thyrotrophin (thyroid stimulating hormone)

With dietary iodine as an essential material

The thyroid gland manufactures and stores:
– Thyroxine (T4), in the greatest amounts
– Tri-iodothyronine (T3)
– Calcitonin

When released into blood circulation, most T4 and T3 travels attached to thyroid binding globulin
Smaller amounts of the hormones travel free or bound to other plasma proteins.

Circulating free T3 and T4 enters cells.
It binds itself to storage proteins, and is utilised slowly according to the demands of the cell.

Tri-iodothyronine is the active hormone of cell metabolism.
Thyroxine needs to be converted to tri-iodothyronine to become active.
This happens in the tissues of the kidneys, muscles and liver.

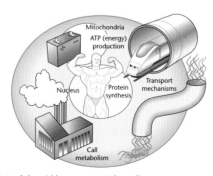

Thyroid gland – the effect of thyroid hormones on the cell

ASSOCIATED INVESTIGATIONS

The results of tests investigating the function of the thyroid gland may be affected by:
- Pregnancy and oral contraceptives
- The acute or convalescent phase of severe illness.

Related pages

Palpation of the thyroid gland	The thyroid gland should be: - Normal in size - Symmetrical - Nodes should not be felt.	
Thyroid stimulating hormone measurement	A raised value, when serum thyroxine is low, indicates hypothyroidism. Decreased levels indicate disease of the hypothalamus or the pituitary gland.	
Serum thyroxine binding globulin	This measures the amount of free binding sites on globulin, available to thyroxine. Levels will rise in hypothyroidism. Levels will lower in hyperthyroidism.	
Thyroid scans: – Iodine or technetium – Ultrasound	These will show the presence of nodes, which can be cysts, or benign or malignant tumours.	
Fine needle biopsy	The aspiration of fluid from a thyroid nodule.	
Haemoglobin	Hypothyroidism will slow the initiation and production of red blood cells, causing anaemia.	38
Pulse rate Respirations	Hyperthyroidism will produce tachycardia and tachypnoea. Hypothyroidism will produce bradycardia and bradypnoea.	9 129

CONSIDERATIONS FOR CARE

The amount of thyroid hormone produced by the thyroid gland will modify the symptoms of disease felt by the patient. Hyperthyroidism and hypothyroidism can vary from subclinical function that produces few effects, to extreme life-threatening conditions. Care must be planned according to the individual experience of each patient.

Both conditions improve when the appropriate therapy has been initiated and thyroid hormone balance is regained.

When a hyperthyroid or hypothyroid patient needs a surgical procedure, care planning must include the maintenance of a correct level of thyroid hormone.

HYPERTHYROIDISM

The thyroid gland is producing too much thyroxine. This is raising the patient's basal metabolic rate above normal. All body processes are becoming more rapid.

A calm, cool, relaxed environment will be needed, to counter the agitation felt by the patient. Activity and stress initiated by the sympathetic nervous system will increase the metabolic rate further.

Speech and thought processes may be rapid to the point of confusion. Time is required for all communications.

An adequate intake of calories will be needed to fuel the increased energy needs. The meals offered should reflect this. Weighing the patient regularly will allow adjustment of the dietary calorific intake against weight loss.

The rapidity of gastrointestinal movement may cause diarrhoea. The patient will need to be situated near a lavatory, to relieve their anxieties about getting to a toilet in time.

The constant nervous agitation will cause increased sweating. Frequent attention to body hygiene will be required.

Sleeping will be difficult for this physically and mentally overactive person. All aids to sleep must be used to help them to rest for as long as they are able.

HYPOTHYROIDISM

The thyroid gland is producing too little thyroid hormone. This is lowering the patient's basal metabolic rate. All body processes become slower.

This will cause a feeling of tiredness and apathy that will affect the patient's ability to take responsibility for elements of his or her own care. Help and encouragement may be needed.

A warm environment and sufficient clothes and bedding are needed to counteract the feeling of chill.

Physical and mental functioning will be slow. Memory will become poor. All communications should be paced according to the patient's ability to understand and remember.

Slow metabolism requires fewer calories, so diet needs to be adjusted to prevent a weight gain.

Dietary roughage should also be included to avoid constipation.

The lower body metabolism will mean that medications will remain in the body for longer periods. Care must be taken when using drugs, i.e. sedation.

Thyroid therapy, when commenced, is for the rest of the patient's life. It should be started with a full explanation of its purpose and a programme of checks organised to monitor its effects.

ALTERED VALUES

RAISED VALUES

Hyperthyroidism
– T3 thyrotoxicosis
– Graves' disease

Increased amounts of thyroid
binding globulin,
see below

Lack of carbohydrate and lipids to
utilise the T3
– Fasting

Reduced available oxygen
– High altitudes
– Chronic obstructive airway disease

Effect of drugs, including:
– Thyroxine

Thyroid binding globulin

Excessive production by the liver
– Metastases
– Viral hepatitis

Hypothyroidism

Pregnancy

LOWERED VALUES

Hypothyroidism
– Myxoedema
– Thyroidectomy

Decreased amounts of thyroid
binding globulin,
see below

Iodine deficiency
– Malnutrition

The elderly

Effect of drugs, including:
– Antithyroid drugs

Thyroid binding globulin

Decreased production by the liver
– Hepatic cirrhosis

Hyperthyroidism

Malnutrition

Protein-losing diseases
– Nephrotic syndrome

Use of protein for metabolism
– Cushing's disease
– Prolonged cortisone therapy
– Stress

THYROXINE (T4)

ALTERED VALUES

RAISED VALUES	LOWERED VALUES
Pituitary tumour secreting increased thyroid stimulating hormone	Hypopituitarism
Hyperthyroidism – Thyrotoxicosis – Graves' disease – Multinodular goitre – Solitary toxic nodule – Thyroiditis – Carcinoma of the thyroid	Hypothyroidism (myxoedema) – Thyroidectomy – Autoimmune disease of the thyroid
Increased iodine intake – Dietary – Drug-induced	Iodine deficiency – Malnutrition
Increased levels of thyroid binding globulin – Pregnancy	Decreased levels of thyroid binding globulin – Liver failure – Cushing's syndrome – Nephrotic syndrome
Obesity	Stress – Following serious illness – Post-operative
	Effect of drugs, including: – Long-term cortisone therapy

Thyroid stimulating hormone	Thyroid stimulating hormone
Hypothyroidism – Myxoedema	Hyperthyroidism Causes listed above
Prescribed thyroxine dose too low	
Prescribed antithyroid drug dose too high	

REFERENCE RANGE

Adult: 135–146 mmol/l

Child: 136–143 mmol/l

Neonate: 133–146 mmol/l

PROCEDURE

Venepuncture.

The specimen should be kept at room temperature.

It should be sent to the laboratories within 2 hours.

The blood sample should not be taken from an arm that has an intravenous infusion in place.

CONTAINER

The specimen container used in this unit is:

PURPOSE

To measure the concentration of sodium circulating in the plasma.

This measurement has no correlation with the level of total body sodium, as sodium exchanges are constantly made between the plasma, tissue fluid and intracellular fluids. It can only give a reflection that a sodium imbalance exists.

Sodium and the water content of the body have a close relationship. Sodium attracts water, as it has a strong osmotic pull. A reduction in tissue sodium will diminish this osmotic pull, and less water will be taken into the tissue fluids.

In health, sodium and water balance is kept by adjusting dietary intake, and the renal excretion of each.

Sodium is a positively charged ion – a cation. The largest proportion of sodium is found in the extracellular fluid, where it is the most abundant positively charged electrolyte.

Sodium is needed:
■ As part of the system that keeps the body in electrical balance
■ For fluid balance
■ For muscle function
■ For acid–base balance.

NORMAL PHYSIOLOGY

Dietary intake of sodium
– Food and drinks
– Added salt to food

Sodium absorbed by the small intestine enters:
– The plasma
– Extracellular fluid
– Intracellular fluids

Sodium provides a major osmotic pull, to attract water to the fluid compartments of the body.

*NORMAL SODIUM LEVEL = NORMAL FLUID VOLUMES
    An increased sodium level = increased fluid volumes
    A decreased sodium level = decreased fluid volumes

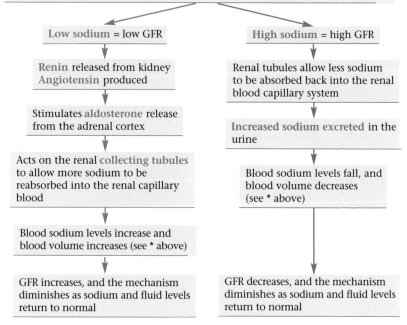

Sodium is taken in the circulating blood to the kidneys
enters the kidney tubules as part of the glomerular filtrate

The amount of sodium taken from the filtrate and reabsorbed into the blood depends on the volume of blood within the renal circulation, measured at the glomerulus (see * above): the glomerular filtration rate or GFR

Low sodium = low GFR	High sodium = high GFR
Renin released from kidney Angiotensin produced	Renal tubules allow less sodium to be absorbed back into the renal blood capillary system
Stimulates aldosterone release from the adrenal cortex	Increased sodium excreted in the urine
Acts on the renal collecting tubules to allow more sodium to be reabsorbed into the renal capillary blood	Blood sodium levels fall, and blood volume decreases (see * above)
Blood sodium levels increase and blood volume increases (see * above)	
GFR increases, and the mechanism diminishes as sodium and fluid levels return to normal	GFR decreases, and the mechanism diminishes as sodium and fluid levels return to normal

Sodium is also lost through the skin and faeces.

ALTERED VALUES

RAISED VALUES	LOWERED VALUES
Hypernatraemia	**Hyponatraemia**

Reduction of circulating volume to dilute the concentration of circulating sodium
Dehydration
– Reduced fluid intake
– Diarrhoea
– Vomiting
– Polyuria, e.g. in:
  – Diabetes mellitus
  – Uraemia
  – Diabetes insipidus
	This usually indicates an excessive loss of sodium rather than poor dietary intake
	Sodium loss from the gastrointestinal tract
	– Aspiration of contents
	– Vomiting
	– Diarrhoea
	– Paralytic ileus

Disorders that initiate the mechanism for sodium to be retained due to changes in the pressure of blood flowing through part or whole of the circulatory system – Hepatic cirrhosis – Nephrotic syndrome – Congestive cardiac failure	Loss from body surface – Draining of ascites – Excessive sweating – Burns
	Loss of sodium through the renal system – Diuretic phase of actue tubular necrosis – Polycystic disease of the kidney
Prolonged intravenous saline infusion therapy	Metabolic disease – Addison's disease, with decreased aldosterone – Hypothyroidism – Acidosis
	Excessive volume of circulating water – Excessive fluid intake, e.g. beer – Oedema
Effect of drugs, including: – Cortisone – Antibiotics	Effect of drugs, including: – Diuretics

ASSOCIATED INVESTIGATIONS

		Related pages
Other electrolytes: ■ Potassium ■ Chloride ■ Bicarbonate	To assess the effect on other electrolytes when sodium values are not within normal limits.	102 107
Blood pH	Sodium moves to maintain correct electrical balance in the tissues, when other electrolytes are used to keep the body pH within normal limits.	150
Tests of kidney function	Presence of sodium-wasting or sodium-retaining disease.	
24-hour urine collection for sodium excretion	The short-term variables that alter sodium excretion will not allow a single random urine specimen to give an accurate estimate of the amount of sodium lost through the kidneys.	
Urine: ■ Osmolality ■ Specific gravity	Both raised when excessive amounts of sodium is excreted.	180
Central venous pressure	Monitors blood volume. Reduced sodium = hypovolaemia. Increased sodium = hypervolaemia.	28
Pulse	Tachycardia develops with hypovolaemia.	9
Blood pressure	Hypovolaemia causes a fall in blood pressure. The renin–angiotensin mechanism decreases the amount of sodium excreted by the kidney.	17
Accurate recording of fluid intake and output	Sodium depletion = loss of body water. Sodium retention = water retention.	
Daily weight	Rapid variations in weight will be attributable to fluid loss or retention. Sodium retention will not allow water (oedema) to leave body tissues.	264 283

CONSIDERATIONS FOR CARE

RAISED VALUES OF BLOOD SODIUM

A raised blood sodium value usually implies a state of dehydration.

An increased fluid intake, to dilute the circulating sodium, will be sufficient to bring the measurement back to normal limits.

When disease is the basis of sodium retention, more active measures are needed.

The retention of water along with the sodium will increase the circulating blood volume. Regular observations of pulse, blood pressure and respirations will be necessary.

The increased body sodium will give the patient a thirst. Fluids should be given as prescribed as appropriate to the causative condition.

There must be strict recording of all fluid intake and output.

Mucous membranes will become dry and sticky. Mouth care will be needed for the patient's comfort, especially if oral fluids can not be offered.

Sodium and water retention in the tissues will cause oedema:
- Skin over the swollen areas will be stretched, and poorly perfused with blood. Pressure area and wound care at these sites will be vitally important.
- Swings in daily weight monitor the loss, or gain, of tissue fluid.

A decrease in dietary sodium may be prescribed. A dietitian should advise.

DECREASED VALUES OF BLOOD SODIUM

When sodium is lost from the body, water is lost at the same time. Replacement sodium and water will be necessary.

Oliguria may be a feature of the decreased circulating fluid volume. A fluid input and output chart will be needed.

The patient may feel lethargic, sick and report a headache. Decreased consciousness will follow, if the condition remains untreated.

Muscles will feel weak and cramp easily. Help will be needed for movement.

Postural hypotension will cause giddiness when standing.

Pulse, blood pressure and respirations should be monitored for warning signs of hypovolaemic shock.

A central venous pressure line may be inserted to determine the degree of hypovolaemia and to prevent an excessive volume of replacement fluid overloading the circulation.

POTASSIUM

REFERENCE RANGE

Adult: 3.4–5.0 mmol/l

Child: 4.1–5.6 mmol/l

Neonate: 4.6–6.7 mmol/l

PROCEDURE

Venepuncture.

Haemolysis of the blood will increase the potassium levels, therefore:
- Do not shake the sample
- Do not refrigerate the blood sample
- If the specimen is not sent to the laboratory promptly, potassium will leak from the cells and raise the plasma potassium.

Do not take blood sample from an arm that has an intravenous infusion in place.

CONTAINER

The specimen container used in this unit is:

PURPOSE

To measure the concentration of potassium circulating in the plasma.

Potassium is a positively charged ion – a cation. It is the most abundant cation found within body cells.

Most body potassium is intracellular, which means that the measurement of extracellular plasma potassium is not a reliable indicator of total body potassium.

Large variations in the quantities of intracellular potassium can occur without causing changes to plasma potassium values.

Potassium constantly moves between intracellular and extracellular fluids, including plasma. Total body potassium must be severely reduced before low plasma potassium values are recorded.

Potassium is needed:
- For transmission of nerve and muscle impulses across cell membranes.
- To maintain the water content of the cell. It has the osmotic pull inside the cell to balance the osmotic pull of sodium outside the cell.
- Through intracellular and extracellular exchanges with hydrogen ions, potassium helps maintain a normal acid–base balance.

Both *raised* or *lowered* potassium values will interfere with the transmission of nerve and muscle impulses to cells, including cardiac and respiratory muscle. If severe, and not reversed, cardiac arrest will follow.

NORMAL PHYSIOLOGY

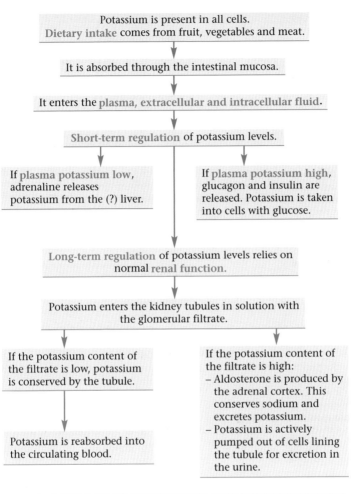

Potassium is present in all cells.
Dietary intake comes from fruit, vegetables and meat.

It is absorbed through the intestinal mucosa.

It enters the plasma, extracellular and intracellular fluid.

Short-term regulation of potassium levels.

If plasma potassium low, adrenaline releases potassium from the (?) liver.

If plasma potassium high, glucagon and insulin are released. Potassium is taken into cells with glucose.

Long-term regulation of potassium levels relies on normal renal function.

Potassium enters the kidney tubules in solution with the glomerular filtrate.

If the potassium content of the filtrate is low, potassium is conserved by the tubule.

Potassium is reabsorbed into the circulating blood.

If the potassium content of the filtrate is high:
– Aldosterone is produced by the adrenal cortex. This conserves sodium and excretes potassium.
– Potassium is actively pumped out of cells lining the tubule for excretion in the urine.

Potassium is also excreted by the skin and in the faeces.
Point of reference:
Alkalosis encourages the movement of potassium from the extracellular fluid into the cells.
Acidosis inhibits potassium from entering cells, pushing intracellular potassium out of the cells and into the extracellular fluid.

ALTERED VALUES

RAISED VALUES	LOWERED VALUES
Hyperkalaemia	**Hypokalaemia**
Excessive potassium intake – Use of salt substitutes – Excessive potassium replacement therapy	Reduced potassium intake – Dietary – Pre-operative starvation – Malabsorption – Prolonged ileus
Tissue damage, releasing potassium from dead and injured cells – Injury or destruction of muscle – Burns – Myocardial infarction	Loss of potassium from the gastrointestinal tract – Vomiting – Nasogastric tube aspiration – Diarrhoea
Movement of potassium out of the cells – Metabolic acidosis – Decreased insulin production	Movement of potassium into the cells – Alkalosis – Insulin-induced hypoglycaemia
Decreased aldosterone production – Addison's disease – Sodium depletion	Increased aldosterone production – Cushing's syndrome – Secondary to other disease, e.g. hypertension
Impaired renal function – Acute renal failure – Severe chronic renal failure – Impaired tubular secretion	Impaired renal function – Following acute tubular necrosis
	Overhydration
	Chronic stress
Effect of drugs, including: – Cytotoxic therapy	Effect of drugs, including: – Insulin – Potassium-wasting diuretics – Bicarbonate – Carbenoxolone sodium

ASSOCIATED INVESTIGATIONS

		Related pages
Pulse	Abnormal levels of body potassium cause cardiac arrhythmias.	9
Electrocardiograph monitoring (ECG)	Raised and lowered levels of potassium produce distinctive features on ECG.	24
Blood pressure	Arrhythmias may lead to a reduction in cardiac output.	17
pH of blood	Alkalosis causes potassium to move from the extracellular fluid into cells. Acidosis causes potassium to leave cells and enter into the extracellular fluid.	150
Respirations	Altered through pH imbalance. Depressed in hyperkalaemia.	129
24-hour urine collection to measure potassium output	The short-term variables that alter potassium excretion will not allow a single random urine specimen to give an accurate estimate of potassium excretion through the kidneys.	
Magnesium	The conditions that reduce blood potassium may also cause a reduction of magnesium. Magnesium speeds the action of enzymes during carbohydrate metabolism. The effect of raised or lowered magnesium values on muscles and nerves gives similar symptoms described when potassium is at abnormal levels.	
Tendon reflexes	Depressed in hyperkalaemia and hypokalaemia.	257

CONSIDERATIONS FOR CARE

The symptoms of a raised or lowered blood potassium are very similar.

In extreme conditions, nerves and muscles are affected to produce:
- Profound weakness, apathy or confusion
- Cardiac arrhythmias.

Sensitive care to accommodate this weakness will be needed. Mobility must be confined to the patient's own limits.

Cardiac involvement needs to be monitored by ECG recordings, pulse and blood pressure. Heart block and cardiac arrest will be possibilities when the condition becomes severe.

Intravenous infusion therapy will be needed to correct both disorders.

Planned care must treat the cause, or the effects, of a raised or lowered potassium state.

HYPERKALAEMIA

The patient may feel tingling and numbness in the face, hands, legs and feet.

Muscle cramps will need to be prevented and eased if they occur.

Nausea and vomiting will initiate the need for good mouth care. Paralytic ileus may develop.

If oral foods are allowed, the diet should be low in potassium. If the high potassium value is a chronic problem, advice on following a low potassium diet and regular medication should be available before discharge from hospital.

HYPOKALAEMIA

The ability of the kidney to concentrate urine will be affected by a low potassium state causing polyuria and thirst. Toilet facilities must be easily available to the patient. Replacement fluids should be given.

Tiredness and apathy are components of this condition and the patient may need help and encouragement with some of the day's events and components of care.

Hazards can arise when potassium is replaced intravenously:
- The potassium must be mixed well into the solution to prevent it concentrating in the container at the site where it was added
- Potassium should not be added to blood or blood products
- The infusion must be slow and controlled
- Potassium should not be given to patients with impaired renal function and for whom the excretion of potassium is difficult.

If appropriate, advice on a high potassium diet should be given before discharge.

REFERENCE RANGE

Adult: 100–106 mmol/l

Child: 98–106 mmol/l

Neonate: 100–117 mmol/l

PROCEDURE

Venepuncture.

CONTAINER

The specimen container used in this unit is:

PURPOSE

To measure the chloride content of the blood plasma.

This can only be a reflection of the total body amount, as most chloride is transported into the extracellular tissue fluid.

Chloride is a negatively charged ion – an anion. As the most abundant anion in the extracellular fluid, it provides an electrical balance to the extracellular cation, sodium.

The main electrolyte partnerships come from:

Chloride (−ve)		Bicarbonate (−ve)
+	=	+
sodium (+ve)		potassium (+ve)
Extracellular		Intracellular

The total number of chloride and bicarbonate anions (negative charge) do not equal the number of sodium and potassium cations (positive charge). This shortfall is made up of small quantities of other negatively charged ions:
- Phosphate
- Sulphate
- Organic ions
- A group of plasma proteins.

Chloride provides:
- An osmotic pressure, for the distribution of extracellular fluid
- An active component for maintaining acid–base balance.

A large amount of chloride is found in the stomach as hydrochloric acid.

As a major purpose of chloride is to keep electrolytes in balance, an abnormal value may signify the abnormal or compensatory movement of other electrolytes.

NORMAL PHYSIOLOGY

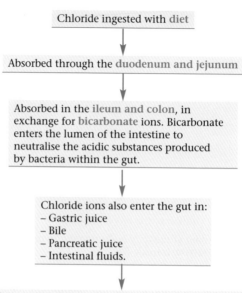

Chloride ingested with diet

Absorbed through the duodenum and jejunum

Absorbed in the ileum and colon, in exchange for bicarbonate ions. Bicarbonate enters the lumen of the intestine to neutralise the acidic substances produced by bacteria within the gut.

Chloride ions also enter the gut in:
– Gastric juice
– Bile
– Pancreatic juice
– Intestinal fluids.

Circulating chloride provides electrical balance with other electrolytes within:
– Plasma
– Cells
– Extracellular fluid

Chloride is taken in the circulating blood to the kidneys, and enters the renal tubules in the glomerular filtrate.

The renal tubules excrete or reabsorb chloride according to the body's need for other electrolytes:
– Chloride is passively reabsorbed when sodium is reabsorbed by the tubule
– Reabsorption of chloride is raised or lowered in opposition to the body's need for **bicarbonate**.

Aldosterone (sodium control) and pH balance (bicarbonate) therefore indirectly influence the excretion of chloride in the urine.

Chloride is also lost through the skin in sweat.

ALTERED VALUES

RAISED VALUES

Hyperchloraemia

Dehydration
Less circulating fluid causes
an increased concentration
of ions
– Diarrhoea

Sodium retention
Causes:
– Hyperaldosteronism
– Congestive cardiac failure
– Acute renal failure

Hyperparathyroidism
Kidneys increase phosphate
output and chloride tries to
maintain anion balance

Metabolic acidosis
The bicarbonate that is
excreted is replaced by
chloride

Respiratory alkalosis

Effect of drugs, including:
– Corticosteroids

LOWERED VALUES

Hypochloraemia

Loss of chloride from the
gastrointestinal tract
– Nasogastric aspiration
– Intestinal obstruction
– Vomiting

Excessive loss of sodium
Causes:
– Addison's disease

Loss through renal tubular damage

Heat exhaustion

Hypokalaemic acidosis
– Decreased potassium levels
  with decreased chloride levels

Respiratory acidosis

Effect of drugs, including:
– Furosemide (frusemide)
– Bendroflumethiazide (bendrofluazide)

ASSOCIATED INVESTIGATIONS

		Related pages
Other electrolytes: ■ Sodium ■ Potassium	Assessment of electrolyte balance.	**97** **102**
pH	When bicarbonate is retained to correct metabolic acidosis, chloride is lost through the kidney.	**150**
Bicarbonate	Bicarbonate is part of the buffering system of the body. It maintains and regulates the pH of the body.	
Respirations	Variations in respirations when the body pH is not correct.	**129**
24-hour urine collection to measure chloride excretion	Chloride is mainly excreted through the kidney.	

CONSIDERATIONS FOR CARE

It is the nature of chloride to counter the imbalances of other electrolytes.

As disease is controlled and electrolytes return to normal, chloride will also return to proper levels.

HYPERCHLORAEMIA

Raised levels of chloride can produce states of weakness.

Adequate help must be given to the patient with all their activities of care.

Levels of consciousness should be monitored.

HYPOCHLORAEMIA

Removal of gastric juice (hydrochloric acid) either by vomiting or continuous aspiration is a common reason for low chloride levels. A fluid intake and output chart should be kept to monitor the gastric aspirate removed, or the number and amounts of vomit.

A regime to replace the lost electrolytes may be commenced.

Movement will need care as the nervous system is irritable and muscles contract into cramps.

Tetany may occur.

CALCIUM

REFERENCE RANGE

Adult: 2.2–2.67 mmol/l

Child: 2.24–2.86 mmol/l

Neonate: 1.5–2.9 mmol/l

PROCEDURE

Venepuncture.

Prolonged use of the tourniquet will cause loss of fluid from the veins into surrounding tissues. This will increase the concentration of plasma proteins in the withdrawn venous blood. As 50% of the plasma calcium travels bound to plasma proteins, the increase in plasma protein will produce an incorrect raised calcium measurement.

CONTAINER

The container used in this unit is:

PURPOSE

To measure the concentration of circulating plasma calcium. Calcium travels in plasma in two ways:
- Without attachment, as an ion. It is in this form that calcium is physiologically active.
- Calcium bound to a plasma protein.
- Complexed calcium.

To fulfil its many functions, calcium is highly mobile. Plasma calcium is the most available way of measuring the calcium balance between bone, tissue, and renal excretion. The mobility of calcium may mean that a single test may give a false representation of true calcium values.

Calcium:
- Gives strength to the skeleton
- Provides interconnections between cells, holding them together
- Maintains the structure and function of cell walls
- Allows sodium to cross cell walls
- Regulates cell metabolism
- Allows conduction of impulses from nerve endings, to stimulate muscle contraction
- Is necessary for blood clotting
- Is an intracellular messenger for hormones.

The multifunctional nature of calcium means that abnormal concentrations of calcium will have many effects. Disordered muscle function may be the most obvious.

A raised calcium concentration will depress the nervous system and cause muscle weakness.

A lowered calcium concentration will lead to overstimulation of muscles by nerve impulses.

This has important implications for cardiac muscle.

NORMAL PHYSIOLOGY

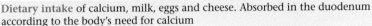

Dietary intake of calcium, milk, eggs and cheese. Absorbed in the duodenum according to the body's need for calcium

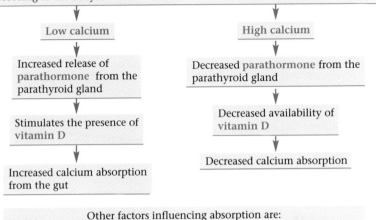

Low calcium

Increased release of parathormone from the parathyroid gland

Stimulates the presence of vitamin D

Increased calcium absorption from the gut

High calcium

Decreased parathormone from the parathyroid gland

Decreased availability of vitamin D

Decreased calcium absorption

Other factors influencing absorption are:
– Pregnancy
– Lactation
– Periods of growth
Calcium present in cells – 99% in bone, extracellular fluid and plasma

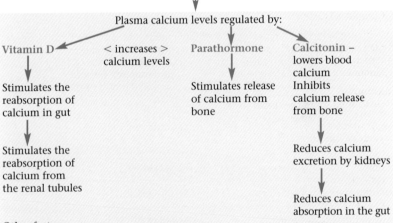

Plasma calcium levels regulated by:

Vitamin D ← increases → calcium levels

Stimulates the reabsorption of calcium in gut

Stimulates the reabsorption of calcium from the renal tubules

Parathormone

Stimulates release of calcium from bone

Calcitonin – lowers blood calcium
Inhibits calcium release from bone

Reduces calcium excretion by kidneys

Reduces calcium absorption in the gut

Other factors:
– Growth hormone retains calcium in bone
– Thyroxine and tri-iodothyronine increase the rate of calcium turnover in bone
– Glucagon suppresses the reabsorption of calcium from bone and releases calcitonin
– Cortisone inhibits calcium reabsorption from bone and increases renal calcium excretion

Calcium in circulating blood is taken to the kidney to be conserved or excreted, according to the above factors. Also some loss in faeces.

ALTERED VALUES

RAISED VALUES	LOWERED VALUES
Hypercalcaemia	**Hypocalcaemia**
	Inadequate intake of dietary calcium
Neoplasms – Tumours that secrete a parathormone-type substance, e.g. carcinoma bronchus – Breakdown of bone from metastases – Multiple myeloma – Plaeochromocytoma	Neoplasms of bone with bone metastases
	Malabsorption of calcium – Rickets – Acute pancreatitis
	Magnesium deficiency
High levels of vitamin D	Vitamin D deficiency – Reduced intake – Malabsorption – Decreased metabolism
Acromegaly	
Paget's disease	
Sarcoidosis	Low albumin levels, to act as a calcium carrier – Nephrotic syndrome
Hyperthyroidism	
Hyperparathyroidism – Hyperplasia – Tumour	Hypoparathyroidism – Congenital causes – Auto-immune causes – Surgical removal of the parathyroid gland
Renal shutdown Excess calcium not secreted	Chronic renal failure
	Renal stones
Immobilisation	Septic shock
Effect of drugs, including: – Vitamin D – Thiazide diuretics – Androgens – Bendroflumethiazide (bendrofluazide)	Effect of drugs, including: – Cytotoxic therapy

ASSOCIATED INVESTIGATIONS

Related pages

Parathormone values	A controlling factor for the absorption and mobilisation of calcium.	
Phosphate values	Normal value: 0.8–1.5 mmol/l. Phosphate and calcium share common control systems. Disruption to calcium metabolism will affect phosphate levels.	
Magnesium values	Normal value: 0.7–1.1 mmol/l. Magnesium is needed for energy production in the cells. It works in opposition to calcium, pacifying rather than activating neuromuscular junctions.	
Serum albumin	50% of circulating calcium is bound to albumin. If albumin values are reduced, there are less vehicles available to carry circulating calcium. Plasma calcium will be reduced.	75
Electrocardiograph recording	Hypocalcaemia causes changes to the ECG tracing.	24
Chvostek's sign	Low calcium concentrations cause the facial nerve to twitch in response to a tap to the nerve, either in front of the temple or on the parotid gland.	
Trousseau's sign	When a sphygmomanometer cuff is placed around the arm and inflated to more than the systolic blood pressure, the forearm muscles begin to twitch when calcium concentrations are low.	

CONSIDERATIONS FOR CARE

HYPERCALCAEMIA

A raised blood calcium may indicate that calcium is being withdrawn from the bones. This weakens bone and pathological fractures are a possibility. This risk must be balanced against the need for the patient to mobilise and exercise. Immobility exacerbates the problem of calcium loss from bone.

Analgesia for bone and joint pain may be needed before movement is attempted. Positioning and movement must be carefully planned and managed.

The combination of a depressed nervous system and muscle weakness will, if untreated, develop into paralysis and unconsciousness.

Recordings of pulse, respirations and blood pressure will be necessary to assess the effect on cardiac function. ECG monitoring may also be recommended.

Adequate food intake must be encouraged as loss of appetite may become a problem.

Discomfort from nausea and vomiting must be properly dealt with. Constipation could also become a problem, if not prevented.

The raised values of plasma calcium may cause calcium deposits to form renal calculi. A high fluid intake is needed to prevent this happening.

HYPOCALCAEMIA

Poor nutrition and lack of vitamin D, as causes of hypocalcaemia, identify the elderly, frail or confined as groups of people at risk from this condition.

Preventative health education and care is therefore extremely important.

Severe hypocalcaemia will cause muscle spasm and tetany. Movement will become painful.

Laryngeal stridor and dyspnoea can develop.

The importance of calcium to cardiac muscle means that a deficiency will induce arrhythmias and heart block. Pulse and blood pressure should be monitored to record changes.

The cause of the deficiency should be investigated and treated.

Calcium replacement therapies must be given.

Intravenous calcium replacement therapy must be delivered slowly, and its effects monitored by an ECG tracing.

REFERENCE RANGE

Blood – Adult: 0.7–1.1 mmol/l

      Child: value is age dependent

      Neonate: 0.6–0.9 mmol/l

PROCEDURE

Venepuncture.

24-hour urine test.

CONTAINER

The specimen container used in this unit is:

PURPOSE

To assess the magnesium content of the blood.

Magnesium is predominantly an intracellular positive ion, with potassium. For this reason there is a minimal amount in the blood for the assessment of total body values of magnesium.

Magnesium is an essential presence when the energy molecule adenosine triphosphate is needed to power intracellular, metabolic processes. Appropriate metabolic cell function also relies on the continuing correct balance of calcium and magnesium availability.

Magnesium is absorbed through the small intestine but a high phosphate diet will reduce this absorption of magnesium. It is transported in the circulating blood to be taken up by the red blood cells, soft tissue and bone. Magnesium balance is maintained through the renal tubules, excreting surplus amounts and reabsorbing back into circulation when magnesium values are reduced.

Magnesium has a calming effect on nerve endings. A surplus of available magnesium, hypermagnesaemia, will increase this effect and depress the activity of the nervous system.

A depletion of magnesium, hypomagnesaemia, will cause nervous hypersensitivity. Symptoms will include tremors, cardiac arrythmias and fits.

ALTERED VALUES

RAISED VALUES	LOWERED VALUES
Rise in ingested magnesium (antacids)	Malnutrition
	Malabsorption Prolonged gastric drainage or diarrhoea
Renal disease, where tubules are unable to excrete excess magnesium	Renal disease, where tubules are unable to conserve magnesium
Addison's disease	Hypercalcaemia
	Diabetic acidosis
	Primary aldosteronism
	Severe burns
	Pregnancy

CREATININE

REFERENCE RANGE

Adult: 60–120 μmol/l

Child: <80 μmol/l

Neonate: 60–120 μmol/l

Values will be higher in the afternoon than the morning.

PROCEDURE

Venepuncture.

Refrigerate specimen if it is not sent immediately to the laboratory.

Room temperature causes the specimen to decay.

CONTAINER

The specimen container used in this unit is:

PURPOSE

To measure the rate of creatinine excretion from the kidneys.

Creatinine is produced as a waste product of anaerobic skeletal muscle metabolism. It is taken to the kidneys for excretion in the urine.

The normal creatinine values will rise according to the muscle mass of the body. For this reason, a man's normal creatinine value will usually be higher than a woman's.

Creatinine values are a good indicator of renal function because:
- The amount of creatinine produced does not vary with dietary intake, although results will be proportional to muscle mass.
- There is a direct link between the amount produced in the muscle and the amount excreted by the kidneys; no other organs are involved to distort the measurements taken.
- Except for a small proportion, which is secreted into the filtrate through the tubule walls, all the creatinine passes through the renal tubule in the glomerular filtrate.

A *raised* blood creatinine value will suggest reduced kidney function, where excretion is unable to keep pace with the creatinine produced by the muscles.

The associated investigations and considerations of care in this circumstance are the same as those applying to a raised blood urea.

A more precise picture of renal function comes from a creatinine clearance test.

A 24-hour urine specimen is taken to see if renal excretion of creatinine correlates with the amount of creatinine produced by the skeletal muscles.

ALTERED VALUES

RAISED VALUES

High red meat diet

Large muscle mass

Reduced blood flow
through the kidneys
– Congestive cardiac failure

Renal disease
– Nephritis
– Renal failure

Acute or chronic obstruction of the
urinary tract
– Renal calculi
– Enlarged prostate

Effect of drugs, including:
– Androgens

LOWERED VALUES

Blood volume expansion
– Pregnancy

Eclampsia

Reduced muscle mass
– Muscular dystrophy

UREA

REFERENCE RANGE

Adult: 2.5–6.7 mmol/l

Child: 2.5–6.7 mmol/l

Neonate: 1.0–8.5 mmol/l

PROCEDURE

Venepuncture.

CONTAINER

The specimen container used in this unit is:

PURPOSE

To measure the concentration of urea circulating in the blood.

Urea is the final waste product of protein metabolism. A proportion of the measured amount is derived from bacteria in the gut and the breakdown of their waste products.

The quantity of urea that appears in the blood depends on:
- The amount of protein taken in the diet
- The amount of protein released when tissue breaks down
- Liver function for urea production
- Degree of hydration
- Renal function, the rate and ability of the nephrons to deal with urea. Renal function has to be reduced by half before there is a rise in blood urea.

Urea is concentrated by the kidneys.

It is not easily reabsorbed back into the circulation through the nephrons.

As an osmotic diuretic, urea attracts water. As urea passes through the nephrons, it takes water through with it, increasing the volume of urine excreted.

Blood urea is an indicator of renal function and hydration, although other factors concerned with the manufacture and excretion of urea will influence the result of the test.

A more accurate assessment of renal function can be made when urea and creatinine clearance results are compared.

NORMAL PHYSIOLOGY

Dietary intake of protein.

↓

Proteins are structures made from chains of amino acids.

↓

Enzymes in the gastrointestinal tract break down the proteins into their amino acid components. The amino acids are absorbed into the blood.

↓

The amino acids are taken to the organs and cells to be re-formed into body proteins, i.e. enzymes, blood cells, hormones. There is a limit to the body's need for amino acids, to replenish its protein requirement.

↓

Excess amino acids are taken to the liver where they are broken down (or degraded) to be either:

- Used for energy
- Stored as fat.

The liver de-aminates the amino acids releasing ammonia.

Ammonia is also produced by the bacteria in the gut.

This is absorbed into the blood circulation and taken to the liver.

In the liver, the ammonia combines with carbon dioxide to produce urea.

↓

The urea is secreted into the blood. It is taken to the kidneys where it enters the renal tubules with the glomerular filtrate.

↓

The osmotic diuretic property of urea increases the volume of water excreted in the urine.

↓

Urea is excreted in the urine.

ALTERED VALUES

RAISED VALUES

High protein diet

Dehydration
– Inadequate fluid intake
– Excessive fluid loss

The use of protein for cell metabolism
– Diabetes mellitus
– Steroid therapy
– Cushing's disease

Increased release of adrenaline
– Stress
– Shock

Extensive tissue destruction
– Gastrointestinal bleeding
– Severe infection
– Necrosis
– Acute phase of auto-immune diseases

Reduced blood flow to kidneys
– Congestive cardiac failure

Renal disease decreasing filtrate flow through tubules
– Pyelonephritis
– Polycystic kidneys

Urinary tract obstruction
– Prostatic enlargement
– Renal calculi

Effect of drugs, including:
– Corticosteroids

LOWERED VALUES

Low protein diet

Very dilute urine
– Diabetes insipidus
– Excessive fluid intake

Increase in blood volume with pregnancy

Liver unable to form urea
– Cirrhosis
– Hepatitis

ASSOCIATED INVESTIGATIONS

		Related pages
Urine testing	To test for abnormal constituents or abnormal measurement of urine components.	174
Fluid input and output chart	To measure urine volume.	
Serum creatinine	A kidney reduced in function can not excrete creatinine produced by the muscles. The value of serum creatinine will rise.	119
Urine creatinine 24-hour collection	Assessment of kidney function by quantifying the ability of the kidney to excrete waste products.	
Electrolyte balance ▪ Sodium ▪ Potassium ▪ Bicarbonate ▪ Chloride	Renal disease will destabilise sodium balance and acid–base balance.	97 102 107
Urea concentration clearance tests	Tests the ability of the kidney to concentrate and excrete urea.	121
Serum calcium Serum phosphate	Renal failure initiates events that disturb the normal process of calcium and phosphate metabolism.	112
Liver function tests	To assess the adequacy of the liver to metabolise protein to produce the end product of urea.	

X-RAY INVESTIGATIONS

Intravenous pylogram	These investigations make observable: ▪ New growths ▪ Obstructions	295
Intravenous urogram	▪ Measurements of the kidney and other structures ▪ Emptying of the bladder	
Cystography	▪ Comparisons between the two kidneys	
Antegrade urography		

SCANS Ultrasound Computerised tomography		298

CONSIDERATIONS FOR CARE

RAISED BLOOD UREA

A high blood urea is termed uraemia or azotemia.

The signs that become associated with a raised blood urea are the consequence of reduced kidney function rather than a direct result of the high blood urea.

The patient may feel weak and tired as anaemia, nerve and muscle weakness become part of the condition. Help must be given to ease the patient through all aspects of their daily care.

Respirations should be monitored. Breathlessness occurs if the patient becomes acidotic. The anaemia and muscle weakness will contribute to this.

Dietary protein intake will need to be reduced. The patient may lose their appetite, feel nauseous or be vomiting. Care should be managed to reduce their discomfort. Prescribed anti-emetics should be available and the patient must be offered appetising food. If the patient is unable to eat, nutrition should be given using other methods.

Fluid intake will be dependent on the ability of the kidney to excrete water. An accurate fluid intake and output chart will be essential.

The patient may be oliguric and need a reduced fluid intake. The skin should be examined for signs of oedema.

The patient may be polyuric, and need large amounts of fluids. Skin and mucous membranes will become dry.

Skin care will be essential to avoid soreness and ulcer formation. Pruritis often develops with uraemia. Application of soothing creams will then be needed.

The mouth can become dry, and have an unpleasant taste. Good regular mouth hygiene will be needed. A fresh mouth will also help when patients are trying to take their diet.

Headache may become severe and analgesia must be available.

Blood pressure should be regularly checked. Hypertension or hypotension may become features of these disorders.

The patient's immune system will be compromised. A rise in the patient's temperature will be significant.

According to the progress of the kidney dysfunction, peritoneal dialysis or haemodialysis may be offered to restore renal homeostasis.

LOWERED BLOOD UREA

If urea is not being formed because of hepatic failure, ammonia accumulates in the blood. This toxic substance will cause unconsciousness and death.

If a low protein diet is the cause of the low urea, the circumstances of this poor quality diet should be explored and dietary help and advice offered.

BLOOD LIPIDS

REFERENCE RANGE

Cholesterol

Adult: 3.5–6.5 mmol/l

Child: 1.8–4.5 mmol/l

PROCEDURE

Venepuncture.

Normal diet and normal health for 2 weeks prior to test.

Water only by mouth 12 hours before the test.

Cell membrane damage from prolonged use of the tourniquet will increase the values.

CONTAINER

The specimen container used in this unit is:

PURPOSE

To assess the lipid content of the blood as cholesterol, triglycerides and fatty acids.

The various structures and transport methods used by blood lipids can be obtained as differentiated blood values.

The results of 2 cholesterol tests, with a minimum of 1 week between, must be known before clinical decisions can be made on the results.

Lipids in their various forms are essential components of cell membranes, required for the formation of bile and steroid hormones, and provide a store of energy.

Cholesterol and triglyceride values are significant to the prevention of heart disease, and the build up of atheromatous plaques in blood vessels.

Lipids are not water soluble. They can only travel in the blood attached to lipo-proteins. It is the classification of four different types of lipoproteins that can categorise cholesterol testing:
- Chylomicrons carry triglycerides
- Very low density lipoproteins (VLDLs) carry triglycerides
- Low density lipoproteins (LDLs) carry cholesterol
- High density lipoproteins (HDLs) carry cholesterol to the liver for elimination. High values of HDLs have a protective effect against coronary heart disease.

NORMAL PHYSIOLOGY

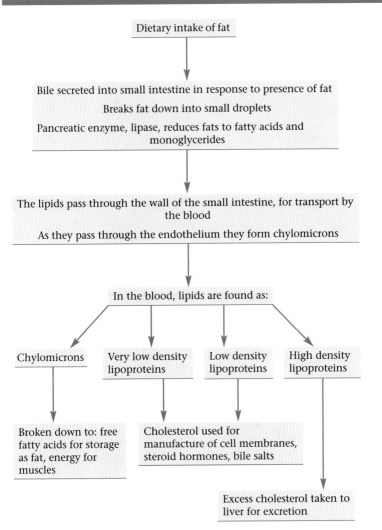

Dietary intake of fat

Bile secreted into small intestine in response to presence of fat

Breaks fat down into small droplets

Pancreatic enzyme, lipase, reduces fats to fatty acids and monoglycerides

The lipids pass through the wall of the small intestine, for transport by the blood

As they pass through the endothelium they form chylomicrons

In the blood, lipids are found as:

Chylomicrons

Very low density lipoproteins

Low density lipoproteins

High density lipoproteins

Broken down to: free fatty acids for storage as fat, energy for muscles

Cholesterol used for manufacture of cell membranes, steroid hormones, bile salts

Excess cholesterol taken to liver for excretion

ALTERED VALUES

RAISED VALUES	LOWERED VALUES
Genetic predisposition to: Hyperlipidaemia	Recent infection
Diabetes mellitus	Malabsorption
Hypothyroidism	Hyperthyroidism
Obstructive jaundice	
Nephrotic syndrome	
Pregnancy	
Alcohol abuse	Drugs: – Oral contraceptives – Salicylates

REFERENCE RANGE

Adult: 14–20 respirations/min

Child: 16–20 respirations/min

Neonate: 30–50 respirations/min

NORMAL CHARACTERISTICS

Respirations should:
- Be at a correct rate
- Have a regular pattern
- Be of equal depth
- Have smooth, easy and symmetrical movements
- Be without noise.

PROCEDURE

It is preferable to count respirations while the patient is distracted. The characteristics of the respirations may alter when they are consciously controlled.

PURPOSE

Respirations ensure that blood gases, especially oxygen and carbon dioxide, remain stable within normal limits.

Inspiration and expiration are the external, measurable signs of the various activities that maintain gas exchanges in balance.

Inspiration brings outside air down through the bronchial tree to provide a new supply of air to the alveoli. Oxygen from the air diffuses through the alveolar wall into the blood.

Oxygen is taken by the blood to the tissues and cells, where it supplies energy for cell function.

Carbon dioxide, a waste product of cell metabolism, diffuses from the tissues into the blood, and is taken back to the lungs. Here it passes back through the capillary wall, into the alveolus.

Expiration pushes air out of the alveolus, expelling the carbon dioxide with it.

The alveoli are not completely emptied of air with every expiration. New air mixes with existing air so that the changes in gas pressures are gradual and blood gases are not swinging to extremes. They are kept in a stable but changing state.

Changes in the rate and character of respirations arise when:
- Disease does not allow an adequate air flow, to or from the alveoli.
- Disease lengthens the distance that gases need to travel from one site to another. The thin alveolar and capillary walls lie in the closest proximity to each other to give gases the shortest, most direct route for diffusion. Disease may cause a thickening of these membranes or fluid formation between the layers.
- The blood is unable to transport sufficient quantities of oxygen or carbon dioxide.

The regulation of the rate of inspiration is controlled by the brain. The respiratory centre responds to changes in the carbon dioxide and oxygen levels of the blood. Respiratory disease will affect it. Other factors that cause blood gases to fluctuate and directly stimulate respiratory activity are exercise, and an increased metabolic rate.

NORMAL PHYSIOLOGY

Respiratory regulation centre
Sited in the medulla oblongata and pons areas of the brain, it is stimulated to alter **rate** and **strength** of respirations by:

1. **Raised blood carbon dioxide concentration.**
   Causes hydrogen ion concentrations to rise in the blood. This directly stimulates the respiratory centre.

2. **Lowered blood oxygen concentrations** and a raised blood carbon dioxide level.
   These are monitored by the carotid bodies in the carotid arteries and aortic bodies in the aortic arch.
   They cause nerve signals to be sent to the respiratory centre.

3. Respirations can also be put under **voluntary control**.

The nerve signals that are sent from the respiratory centre begin weakly and gradually become stronger.

This makes the respiration a slower steadier process, when the lungs are expanding.

Inspiration: an active process, muscles are required to stretch.
- The diaphragm is pulled downwards
- The ribs are pulled outwards and upwards.

Inspiration causes the air pressure of the alveoli to be lower than the outside air.

Air is drawn into the nose passing down to the alveoli to try to equalise the air pressures.

The nose and respiratory passages, with their covering of mucus, warm and humidify the incoming air; their lining of cilia filters and ejects solid particles.

Inspiratory movement ends when:
- The respiratory centre switches off the nervous stimulation
- Sensors in the respiratory tract become overstretched
- Air enters the **alveoli**.

Oxygen passes into the capillary blood surrounding the alveolus
▼
Oxygen travels in the blood to the body tissues and cells
▼
Oxygen and carbohydrates together provide the energy and fuel for cell function
▼
Carbon dioxide and water are the waste products of this process
▼
Carbon dioxide diffuses into the capillary blood, to be taken to the lungs for excretion during expiration.

Expiration is the passive recoil of muscles that follows each active inspiration.

The sudden reduction of space within the thoracic cavity raises the air pressure in the alveoli, above external air.

Alveolar air is pushed up through the respiratory tract, for expulsion through the nose and mouth.

FACTORS AFFECTING NORMAL RESPIRATION

Respirations will become abnormal in character when disease or dysfunction interfere with these five major respiratory processes.

Regulation of the respiratory centre in the brain.
- A raised or lowered blood carbon dioxide concentration causing an altered blood pH
- A lowered blood oxygen concentration
- Conscious respiratory effort and control
- Tumour or damage to the brain stem
- Drugs that depress the respiratory centre, e.g. opiates.

The transmission of nerve impulses between the respiratory centre and the lungs.
- Degeneration of the nerve fibres, e.g. multiple sclerosis
- Injury to the nerve fibres
- Inflammation of the nerve fibres
- Disorders of the neuromuscular junction, e.g. myasthenia gravis.

The muscular expansion of the thoracic cage for the inspiration of air.
- Muscle wasting disease
- Stiffness of the lung tissue or rib cage
- Pain through trauma or surgery
- Air, blood or pleural effusion occupying intrathoracic space preventing full lung expansion.

The flow of inspired air through the air passages.
- Obstruction by tongue or foreign object
- Tumours
- Bronchospasm, narrowing the respiratory passages
- Swelling of mucous membrane or surrounding tissues
- Bronchial plugs of mucus or blood
- Oversecretion of the mucous secreting glands due to infection or inflammation
- Damaged collapsed lung tissue
- Neonatal respiratory distress syndrome, causing alveolar collapse.

The gas exchange between the alveolar walls and the capillary blood vessels.
- Increased thickness of alveolar walls
- Pulmonary oedema
- Decreased areas of normal lung tissue for gaseous exchange
- Decreased amount of available haemoglobin to pick up the oxygen
- Slow or inadequate blood supply to the lungs for sufficient diffusion of oxygen and carbon dioxide across the membrane.

ABNORMAL CHARACTERISTICS

BREATHLESSNESS

The patient may report variations in the type of breathlessness experienced.
Considerations when assessing breathlessness:
- The frequency and duration of the breathless episode
- The distress it causes the patient
- Sounds made by the respirations
- Breathlessness causing a change in skin colour
- Events or actions that initiate the breathlessness
- Lack of breath may interrupt the patient's speech
- A breathless infant will find feeding difficult and tiring.

TACHYPNOEA

Rapid respirations.

Normal response to an increased demand for oxygen:
- Exercise
- Increased metabolism.

Increased stimulus to the respiratory regulation centre:
- Increased carbon dioxide concentrations, lowering the blood pH
- Lowered blood oxygen values.

HYPERPNOEA

An increase in the rate and depth of respiration.

This increases the rapidity and volume of air entering the lungs, when gaseous
exchanges in the alveoli need to be accelerated.

HYPERVENTILATION

Overbreathing.

The marked increase in depth and rate of respirations.
This may be under conscious control.

Psychological disturbances, e.g. stress and panic attacks, may precipitate
hyperventilation.

DYSPNOEA

Breathlessness.

The patient becomes breathless in situations that would not normally be
considered sufficient to cause breathlessness. This may or may not be associated
with exertion.

ORTHOPNOEA

Breathlessness when lying down.

Lying down causes pulmonary congestion and the abdominal organs to push up
against the diaphragm, reducing the capacity of the lungs to expand.

PAROXYSMAL NOCTURNAL DYSPNOEA

Woken from sleep by a sudden onset of breathlessness.

Pulmonary oedema collects while the patient is lying asleep. It causes them to
wake suddenly, distressed and fighting for breath.

PAIN ASSOCIATED WITH INSPIRATION OR EXPIRATION

Abnormal respiratory patterns

Cheyne Stokes respirations
Infrequent slow inspiration, followed by muscle recoil, causing expiration followed by a period of apnoea.

It is a serious sign in the terminally ill.

Kassmaul's respirations
Deep, sighing respirations.
Severe states of acidosis.

Abnormal respiratory sounds

Wheeze
Air is obstructed in the respiratory passages during expiration.

Stridor
Sound of respiratory effort during inspiration.

Stertorous respirations
Noises made by movement of secretions during respirations, or when snoring.

Respiratory movement

Abnormal-shaped chest
Bone disease may affect the shape of the rib cage and its ability to expand for inspiration.

Weak or lack of respiratory movement
Movement of the chest wall may be reduced or absent due to muscle weakness or shallow breathing.

The movements of the rib cage should be symmetrical.

Lack of movement one side may be due to:
- Trauma to the ribs
- Trauma to the lung
- Pain.

The use of chest or abdominal muscles to aid lung expansion and increase the amount of air taken in during inspiration.

Signs of poor oxygenation

Skin colour
When blood is not picking up sufficient oxygen across the alveolar wall, the rise in deoxygenated haemoglobin will cause skin and mucous membranes to colour blue.

Central cyanosis: blueness to the mouth and lips.

Peripheral cyanosis: blueness to the skin and fingernails.

Reduced blood flow will give the appearance of cyanosis even if the blood is fully oxygenated.

Clubbing of the finger tips
Long-term lack of oxygen to the finger tips cause the finger tips to enlarge and the nails to become ridged.

Abnormal characteristics

Respiratory secretions

Nasal secretions

Causes:

Irritants
- Occurs when in contact with allergen
- Often a constant watery discharge
- May come at same time each year.

Infections
- Thicker mucus
- May have green or yellow colour
- May become bloodstained.

Polyps
- Condition does not improve.

Neoplasms
- May be bloodstained
- Nose may feel blocked
- May lose sense of smell.

Sputum
The production of sputum can be caused by:
- Infections
- Inflammations
- Neoplasms
- Pulmonary oedema.

Characteristics of the sputum should be noted:
- Colour
- Amount produced
- Presence of blood
- Frothy sputum associated with pulmonary oedema.

Cough
A cough can be a sign of:
- Infection
- Inflammation
- Neoplasm
- Psychological discomfort.

The characteristics to note about a cough are:
- Whether it is a dry-sounding cough or secretions are moved by its force – productive or non-productive of sputum
- Known factors initiating it
- Its regularity – occasional or persistent
- Length of time the coughing takes – single cough or a prolonged fit of coughing
- Whether the cough is painful
- Whether the noise of the cough is suggestive of a condition, e.g. a whoop with whooping cough or the bark of croup.

ASSOCIATED INVESTIGATIONS

		Related pages
Temperature	Will be raised in the presence of infection.	4
Specimens for culture	Throat swab, sputum, nasopharyngeal aspirate.	294
Full blood count	Amount of available haemoglobin for oxygen uptake. Increase in white cells when inflammation or infection are present.	38 44
Electrolyte monitoring	Disturbance of blood gases and pH values will cause imbalance of electrolytes.	
Arterial blood sampling for:	■ Blood gases – Assess gaseous exchange across the alveolar membrane. ■ Blood pH – States of acidosis and alkalosis will alter the rate and depth of respirations.	
Gas transfer factor	Measures carbon monoxide transfer across the alveolar wall.	
Auscultation and percussion of the chest	Entry of air into lungs, non-functioning areas of the lungs, respiratory noises.	
Chest X-ray	Shows the position and shape of the organs. Shadowing or abnormal lung picture.	295
Pulmonary angiography	Radio-opaque medium from a catheter feeding the pulmonary circulation gives detailed picture of the pulmonary blood vessels.	
Bronchial angiography	A detailed picture of the bronchial arteries.	
Oxygen saturations	Measures the amount of oxygen uptake by the haemoglobin.	142
Skin sensitivities	Tests to identify allergens that cause respiratory problems.	
Cytology	Sputum, following ■ Bronchoscopy ■ Laryngoscopy ■ Removal of pleural aspirate.	
Lung function tests	Measurement of specified gas volumes in the lungs. Peak expiratory flow rate – the amount of air flow on expiration. Spirometry – measures the rate of air flow expired against a time scale. Lung volume measurement – measures the total thoracic gas volume.	
Lung scans ■ Perfusion lung scans ■ Ultrasound scans ■ Computerised tomography ■ Magnetic resonance imaging	Indicates the presence of neoplasms. Indicates the distribution of blood flow through the lungs.	
Fibre optic bronchoscopy	Gives direct vision and access for tissue biopsy.	
Pleural aspirations	A sample of pleural fluid taken from pleural effusion.	

CONSIDERATIONS FOR CARE

Breathing is fundamental to life. When breathing becomes difficult, it is frightening for the patient and for their family. Restlessness and agitation may become part of the condition, generating stress, and making the situation worse. These patients and their families will need to be cared for by confident, competent staff in a calm environment.

Communication may be difficult as breathlessness can interrupt speech. The inability to make themselves understood will increase anxiety. Patience will be needed to allow the patients to express themselves properly.

Sitting the patient in a position that will help lung expansion may help. They must also feel comfortable, safe and sufficiently well supported to give them a restful sleep.

Medication, when given, must be assessed for effectiveness to relieve respiratory symptoms.

If nebulisers or nebuhalers are prescribed, they must be prepared, used and cleaned correctly.

Humidified air may be helpful.

Oxygen therapy is discussed on page **146**.

Coughing and expectoration can be uncomfortable but, when mucus is causing obstruction to the flow of air through the lungs, it must be encouraged. Physiotherapy will help, although it is not always welcomed by the patient.

Other helping measures will include:
- Mobilisation to the extent of the patient's ability, without causing exhaustion
- A good fluid intake – dehydration will make the secretions difficult to move
- Hot drinks are often soothing
- Fluids may be restricted if pulmonary oedema is a problem.

Chewing and swallowing when short of breath is difficult. The diet must be adapted to the patient's ability to eat and to the foods that they find appetising. The diet should contain sufficient roughage to avoid constipation. Bowel preparations should be given if the diet has no effect, as the exertion of straining at stool must be avoided.

Breathless infants find sucking and feeding difficult. If finishing a complete bottle feed becomes difficult, the remaining milk can be given through a nasogastric tube.

An apnoea alarm will give immediate warning that breathing has stopped.

Breathing with the mouth open to increase air intake will make the mucous membranes dry. Mouth care should be given to keep the mouth moist and fresh.

Suction is unpleasant for the patient and a potentially hazardous way of removing respiratory secretions. If it must be done, local policies and procedures need to be followed.

PEAK EXPIRATORY FLOW RATE

NORMAL MEASUREMENT

The normal peak expiratory flow rate has to be calculated for each patient.

The normal calculated value will depend on the patient's age, sex and height.

Measured results need to be plotted against a graph based on criteria pertinent to the patient, i.e. male, female or child.

The measured maximum velocity of expired air is considered normal when it is:
■ Equal to the patient's own known value
■ Within the normal parameters set down by the appropriate graph.

PROCEDURE

Measurement of peak expiratory flow rate will need to be carried out according to local policy, procedure and manufacturer's instructions that accompany the measuring meter.

The accuracy of this test will depend on the patient's competence when using the peak flow meter. The test is inappropriate for young children who are unable to understand instruction.

Explanation and time will be needed for the patient to perfect the technique:
■ To get maximum inspiration
■ To seal the lips tightly around the mouthpiece of the meter
■ The peak flow meter must be held horizontally
■ Of maximum rapid exhalation into the mouthpiece of the peak flow meter.

Three measurements are taken and the highest is plotted on the graph.

Twin measurements recording the peak expiratory flow may be taken while lying, then standing.

PURPOSE

To measure the maximum velocity of air flow during a forced expiration.

This test depends on:
■ The lungs' ability to fill with the correct amount of inspired air
■ The ability of the respiratory muscles to expire air from the lungs with force
■ Patent airways that allow expected volumes of air to be expired.

This test is useful:
■ To monitor respiratory disease during the acute phase
■ Following medication for respiratory disorder, an improvement in peak expiratory flow rates would establish the effectiveness of the treatment
■ To show respiratory sensitivities and allergic response following exposure to suspect materials
■ To chart changes in respiratory capabilities that follow a daily or seasonal pattern.

Decreased peak flow patterns will be seen when:
■ Respiratory muscles are weak
■ There is obstruction to the flow of expired air
■ There is bronchoconstriction.

The total capacity of the lungs for inspired air – Inspiratory capacity =

- Tidal volume, V_T → The volume of air expelled during normal expiration
- + Inspiratory reserve volume → The additional amount of air that can be inhaled with further inspiratory effort.

The total capacity of the lungs – TLC =

- The inspiratory capacity → See above
- + The residual volume → The volume of air remaining in the lungs after forced expiration.

The maximum volume of air that can be exhaled after a maximum inhalation – Forced vital capacity, FVC =

- The inspiratory volume → Air filling the inspiratory capacity becomes the inspiratory volume
- + Tidal volume → See above (V_T)
- + Expiratory reserve volume → The amount of air that remains in the lungs after a normal expiration but can be removed by further forced expiration.

Timed vital capacity, FEVT =

- The volume of air that can be expelled from the lungs, timed at one second (FEV_1), two seconds (FEV_2) and three seconds (FEV_3). The results are expressed as a percentage of the measured vital capacity.

The amount of air remaining in the lungs after normal expiration – Functional residual volume, FRC =

- Expiratory residual volume → See above
- + The residual volume → See above

REFERENCE RANGE

Arterial PO_2: 10–13.3 kPa or 75–100 mmHg

Arterial PO_2 (Neonate): 7–10 kPa or 60–80 mmHg

PROCEDURE

Measurement from arterial blood:
- Arterial stab
- Arterial cannulation.

Apply pressure to puncture site for at least 5 min to prevent further bleeding or bruising.

The specimen must not be exposed to the air.

The specimen must be analysed immediately.

CONTAINER

- Capillary tube
- Syringe.

PURPOSE

Arterial blood oxygen is measured to ensure that an adequate supply of oxygen is available to the tissues for metabolism.

Inhaled air contains a variety of gases.

Of the various gas percentages, oxygen measures about 21% of the total gas volume, 19.5% in humidified air.

The movement of oxygen in the body depends on pressures. Oxygen will always move (or diffuse) from an area of high pressure of oxygen to an area of lower oxygen pressure. This movement will be an attempt to make the pressure of oxygen equal in both places. It may be termed as 'the oxygen cascade', as oxygen always travels down a pressure gradient.

The purpose of oxygen is to fuel energy production, for cell metabolism.

It is processed in the mitochondria of the cell, with available nutrients, i.e. glucose, to produce energy or adenosine triphosphate (ATP). The energy produced permits cells to live and do their work.

To produce energy in the correct amounts, oxygen must be delivered to the cells:
- In the right quantity
- At the right rate.

A deficiency in arterial oxygen levels may indicate:
- Too little oxygen reaching the alveoli of the lungs from the air
- Inadequate oxygen diffusion between the alveolus and capillary blood
- Inadequate means of transport for oxygen in the blood
- The inability of tissues to use the oxygen.

A seriously decreased arterial concentration of oxygen will deprive cells of a fundamental energy source. If the condition remains uncorrected, tissue damage and death will occur.

NORMAL PHYSIOLOGY

Air containing oxygen is breathed in during **inspiration**.

The amount breathed in depends on:
- The percentage of oxygen in the inspired air
- The rate and depth of respirations.

The rate and depth of the respirations are controlled by the **respiratory centre** in the brain.

This centre is stimulated primarily by the effects of increased carbon dioxide in the blood.

A lack of oxygen will indirectly activate the centre.

The fresh supplies of oxygen mix with the oxygen that remained in the alveoli after the previous expiration. This mixing ensures that the supplies of oxygen are continuous and stable, and avoids swings in the availability of oxygen.

Oxygen in the alveoli air is at a higher pressure than oxygen in the blood capillaries that surround the alveolus, therefore:

Oxygen diffuses down the pressure gradient out of the alveolus into the capillary blood.

The **alveolar wall** and the **blood capillary** have very thin walls and lie very close together to minimise the diffusing distance.

The oxygen is picked up by the red blood cells in the pulmonary capillary blood vessels. Capillary blood vessels are very narrow at the alveolus and the red blood cells touch the capillary walls. This reduces the diffusing distance, and oxygen passes easily through plasma before reaching its transport molecule, haemoglobin in the red blood cell.

Oxygen combines loosely with the haemoglobin to form **oxyhaemoglobin**.

Oxygen is carried in the blood to the tissues where the oxygen pressures are lower than the pressure in the capillary, therefore:

Oxygen diffuses down the pressure gradient into the tissues.

As oxygen is utilised in the cells for energy production, the pressure of oxygen in the cells falls lower than the pressure in the surrounding tissues. This initiates the continuing diffusion of oxygen down the pressure gradient into the cell.

Oxygen and glucose are used by the cell mitochondria to create energy.

This energy is used to power the processes of cell metabolism.

ALTERED VALUES

RAISED BLOOD VALUES	LOWERED BLOOD VALUES
	Hypoxia
High concentration of oxygen in inspired air	Low concentration of oxygen in inspired air – High altitude
Hyperventilation	Hypoventilation – Obstruction of the airway – Neck position – Head injury – Thoracic injury – Drugs that depress the respiratory centre – Neuromuscular disorders
Hyperbaric oxygen therapy	
	Inadequate delivery of oxygen to the alveolar blood capillaries – Increased diffusing distance, thickened tissue – Fluid between alveolar wall and capillary wall – Ineffective or collapsing alveoli
	Poor oxygen transport from lungs to tissues – Anaemia – Abnormal haemoglobin – Poor circulation of blood, acute or chronic – Local vascular disorders in the lungs or in the tissues
	Tissues unable to use available oxygen – Poisoning, e.g. cyanide – Beriberi
	Atrioventricular shunts – Atrial septal defect – Ventricular septal defect
	Patent ductus arteriosus

OXYGEN SATURATION MONITORING

REFERENCE RANGE

95%–99% oxygen saturation (SaO_2)

PROCEDURE

Measured with a pulse oximeter.

The literature that accompanies each oximeter should be read to ensure that each make of machine is being used correctly.

Some common principles apply to obtain a correct oxygen saturation measurement:
- Time must be given for the measurement to stabilise, between attaching the monitor to the skin and reading the recorded oxygen saturation on the machine.
- The part of the body where the probe is attached must be kept warm and well supplied with blood.
- A good secure contact must be kept between the probe and the skin.
- A bright light shining on the probe will give a false reading.

PURPOSE

To assess the percentage of arterial haemoglobin that is saturated with oxygen.

The act of inspiration brings a fresh supply of oxygen to the lungs. Oxygen diffuses through the alveolar wall into the pulmonary capillaries where it combines with haemoglobin, in the red blood cells. It is haemoglobin molecules that carry oxygen to the tissues. Pressure differences continue to move oxygen from the blood to the tissues, where it provides a fuel for cell function.

Each haemoglobin molecule is designed to pick up four molecules of oxygen. As oxygen combines with the available sites on the haemoglobin, it is that the molecule is becoming 'saturated'. When all the available sites on the haemoglobin have oxygen attached, the haemoglobin molecules are at their maximum saturation of 99%.

The presence of oxygen turns the blue haemoglobin into red oxyhaemoglobin. The degree of 'redness' indicates the degree of oxygen saturation, and it is this that the oxygen saturation monitor measures. It is a non-invasive, simple procedure that gives an alarm when inadequate oxygen is available for use by the tissues.

Oxygen saturation monitoring is useful:
- To monitor the status of oxygen perfusion when disease is present
- When oxygen therapy is in progress. The percentage of given oxygen can be adjusted according to the saturation levels recorded, to maintain normal oxygen saturation values.

A *fall* in oxygen saturation levels will occur when:
- Insufficient oxygen is diffusing through the alveolar wall to saturate the haemoglobin fully
- An abnormality of the haemoglobin does not allow it to become fully saturated.

NORMAL PHYSIOLOGY

Inspired air contains fresh supplies of oxygen. The air is drawn down to the alveoli of the lungs during **inspiration**.

Oxygen diffuses down a pressure gradient, through the alveolar wall and enters the blood capillaries that surround the alveolus.

Oxygen is picked up by the haemoglobin in the red blood cells.

1 haemoglobin molecule = 4 molecules of oxygen = maximum saturation

The haemoglobin/oxygen attachment is loose, allowing easy separation of the oxygen from the haemoglobin, at the tissues.

The relationship between the varying pressures of oxygen in the blood and tissues, and the given pressure at which oxygen becomes attached to or separates from haemoglobin, is described by the **oxygen dissociation curve**.

When pressures of available oxygen are plotted on a graph against the percentage of oxygen attached to haemoglobin it can be seen that even when a maximum amount of oxygen is available to be attached to a maximum amount of haemoglobin, the oxygen saturation levels only reach 97%–99%. It is the presence of carbon dioxide that prevents haemoglobin achieving 100% oxygen saturation.

The affinity between oxygen and haemoglobin does alter under some circumstances.

A reduced affinity for oxygen by haemoglobin means that oxygen is not picked up as easily from the lungs but oxygen is off-loaded more quickly in the tissues. This happens when there is:
- A rise in carbon dioxide concentrations, with its associated acidosis
- A rise in body temperature
- Hypoxia
- Exercise.

An increased affinity for oxygen means that the haemoglobin picks up oxygen more easily at the lungs but requires lower values of oxygen in the tissues before the haemoglobin releases its transported oxygen. This happens when there is:
- A decrease in carbon dioxide values, with its associated alkalosis
- Hypothermia
- Foetal haemoglobin in the blood.

ALTERED VALUES

INCREASED OXYGEN SATURATION	DECREASED OXYGEN SATURATION
100%	**Below 95%**
High concentrations of oxygen in inspired air	Low concentrations of oxygen in inspired air – High altitudes
Hyperbaric oxygen	Hypoventilation – Obstruction of the airways – Neck position – Head injury – Thoracic injury – Drugs that depress the respiratory centre – Neuromuscular disorders
	Inadequate delivery of oxygen to the alveolar blood capillaries – Increased defusing distance, thickened tissue – Fluid between the alveolar wall and the capillary wall – Ineffective or collapsing alveolus
	Disorders of haemoglobin – Carbon monoxide poisoning – Severe anaemia
Increased haemoglobin affinity for oxygen – Lowered carbon dioxide levels and alkalosis, e.g. hyperventilation	Decreased haemoglobin affinity for oxygen – Raised carbon dioxide values and acidosis, e.g. hypoventilation
Hypothermia	Hyperthermia
Abnormal haemoglobin – Foetal haemoglobin – Carboxyhaemoglobin from smoking, gives a false high result	Disorders of the haemoglobin – Carbon monoxide poisoning – Severe anaemia
	Exercise

ASSOCIATED INVESTIGATIONS

		Related pages
Pulse	The pulse rate will indicate the efforts of the heart to distribute the available oxygen to the tissues. The pulse rate will increase when blood is insufficiently oxygenated.	9
Respirations	The respiration rate will increase when there are difficulties maintaining adequate blood values of oxygen.	129
Oxygen saturation measurement	The maintenance of normal oxygen saturation values will be evidence of the effectiveness of oxygen therapy.	142
Accessory muscles of respiration	The use of additional muscles to assist inspiration and expiration should diminish if oxygen therapy improves blood oxygenation.	
The colour and the feel of the skin	The presence of cyanosis is a sign that the blood is insufficiently oxygenated. Damp, cold, white skin is indicative of a shutdown of blood capillary vessels to conserve all available oxygen for the vital organs.	269
Blood gas analysis	Before and during oxygen therapy, the arterial value of:	
	■ Oxygen	139
	■ Carbon dioxide	147
	■ pH	150
	■ Bicarbonate should be known. This will determine: ■ The percentage of oxygen prescribed ■ Its effectiveness as a treatment.	

CONSIDERATIONS FOR CARE

Oxygen therapy should always be used with caution. The percentage of additional, inspired oxygen must be monitored against the measured, circulating oxygen. Only sufficient oxygen to regain and retain normal blood oxygen values should be given.

- Oxygen therapy may diminish the respiratory drive of patients with an increased circulating carbon dioxide.
- Prolonged high values of unmonitored inspired oxygen may produce hyperoxia. Hyperoxia, especially following a period of hypoxia, will cause the release of oxygen free radicals into cells. These will damage and destroy cells, defeating the original purpose of oxygen therapy as a beneficial treatment.
- Oxygen as a combustible gas is a fire hazard. Any materials likely to spark or cause a flame must be kept away from the area of treatment.

A frequent record must be kept of the amount of oxygen given:

- As a percentage in air and
- As litres per minute.

A frequent record must also be kept showing the effectiveness of the treatment:

- Pulse rate
- Respiration rate
- Circulating blood oxygen values, using oxygen saturation monitoring, transcutaneous oxygen monitoring
- The presence of other indicators of respiratory distress.

There are many ways of giving oxygen therapy. The method of choice will depend on the age of the patient, the condition to be treated, and the personal requirements that will bring comfort and relief to each patient.

Putting a mask over the face of a person already in respiratory distress may make them feel even more suffocated, and increase their panic and respiratory efforts. Hold the mask to the face for a short while until they feel confident that they can still breathe with the mask in place.

The oxygen appliances need to be placed correctly, comfortably and securely in position.

Connecting tubing must be supported so that its weight does not drag the appliance out of place and the patient is free to change position.

Keep the skin under the mask dry and comfortable.

Keep the air passages patent for the flow of oxygen by encouraging the removal of mucus by nose blowing and coughing. Physiotherapy will help by loosening secretions and their expectoration. If the patient is unable to co-operate to achieve this, suction will be needed.

It is difficult to speak or eat using an oxygen mask, and respiratory distress may exacerbate these difficulties. To avoid frustration and build the co-operation in care, the patient must not be hurried in either respect.

Sucking feeds may be difficult for babies with oxygen appliances in place. Nasogastric tube feeding can supplement oral feeds or provide an alternative for a short time.

Oxygen has a drying effect on the mucous membranes. This is especially true when oxygen is given through a nasal cannula. Humidifying the oxygen will help. Oral fluids may be increased if the patient's condition permits it.

REFERENCE RANGE

Adult: 4.8–6.1 kPa or 36–46 mmHg

Neonate: 4.8–6.1 kPa or 36–46 mmHg

PROCEDURE

Measurement from arterial blood:
- Arterial stab
- Arterial cannulation.

Apply pressure to the puncture site for at least 5 min to prevent further bleeding or bruising.

The specimen must not be exposed to air.

The specimen must be analysed immediately.

CONTAINER

Capillary tube.

Syringe.

PURPOSE

To measure the carbon dioxide content of the blood.

Carbon dioxide is the waste product formed when energy is metabolised by the cells. It is excreted from the body by the lungs during expiration.

It is the carbon dioxide content in the body that regulates the depth and rate of respirations. Because of this control, carbon dioxide is normally excreted at the same rate as it is formed.

It is the regulation of blood carbon dioxide that maintains the normal pH balance of the blood.

If carbon dioxide rises above normal blood values, the pH value lowers and the body becomes more acidotic.

If, through hyperventilation, blood carbon dioxide values decrease, the pH value rises and the body becomes more alkaline.

The movement of carbon dioxide as a gas relies on pressure differences. It moves from areas where it is at a higher pressure to adjoining areas where the carbon dioxide is at a lower pressure. It moves down a pressure gradient from the cells where it is formed, to the blood, then from the blood to the alveolus for expulsion.

For transport in the blood, carbon dioxide combines with other blood components and takes on other forms. This decreases the amount of free carbon dioxide available to combine with the body water to form acidic carbonic acid, and the body pH remains stable.

An increase in the measured carbon dioxide will indicate either:
- An increase in the amount of carbon dioxide being produced and excreted into the blood, or
- There is a delay in the removal of carbon dioxide from the blood, at the alveoli of the lungs.

NORMAL PHYSIOLOGY

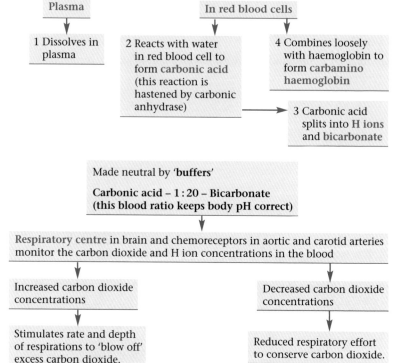

Carbon dioxide produced in cells
as a waste product of energy production.
Carbon dioxide travels down a pressure gradient out of the cell and
enters the blood.
It is transported in the blood in four ways:

Plasma

In red blood cells

1 Dissolves in plasma

2 Reacts with water in red blood cell to form carbonic acid (this reaction is hastened by carbonic anhydrase)

4 Combines loosely with haemoglobin to form carbamino haemoglobin

3 Carbonic acid splits into H ions and bicarbonate

Made neutral by 'buffers'

Carbonic acid – 1:20 – Bicarbonate
(this blood ratio keeps body pH correct)

Respiratory centre in brain and chemoreceptors in aortic and carotid arteries monitor the carbon dioxide and H ion concentrations in the blood

Increased carbon dioxide concentrations

Decreased carbon dioxide concentrations

Stimulates rate and depth of respirations to 'blow off' excess carbon dioxide.

Reduced respiratory effort to conserve carbon dioxide.

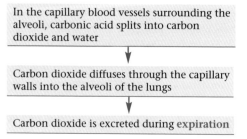

In the capillary blood vessels surrounding the alveoli, carbonic acid splits into carbon dioxide and water

Carbon dioxide diffuses through the capillary walls into the alveoli of the lungs

Carbon dioxide is excreted during expiration

ALTERED VALUES

RAISED VALUES

Hypercapnia

Poor blood circulation back to lungs
– Congestive cardiac failure

Inadequate pulmonary blood
circulation
– Ventricular septal defect
– Atrial septal defect
– Patent ductus arteriosus

Poor diffusion through capillary and
alveolar wall
– Pleurisy
– Pneumonia
– Pulmonary oedema

Inadequate exchange of air during
expiration
– Emphysema
– Asthma
– Hyaline membrane disease

Difficulty with expiration
– Painful expirations
– Neuromuscular weakness

Hypoventilation
– Metabolic alkalosis
– Respiratory acidosis
– Respiratory failure

Electrolyte disturbances
– Severe vomiting

LOWERED VALUES

Hypocapnia

Hyperventilation
– High altitudes
– Metabolic acidosis
– Respiratory alkalosis
– Fever
– Diabetic ketoacidosis

pH BALANCE

REFERENCE RANGE

Arterial blood pH: 7.35–7.45

or

36–45 nanomoles of hydrogen ions per litre of blood (36–45 nmol/l)

PROCEDURE

Measurement from arterial blood:
- Arterial stab
- Arterial cannulation.

Apply pressure to the puncture site for at least 5 min to prevent further bleeding or bruising.

The specimen must not be exposed to air.

The specimen must be analysed immediately.

If carbon dioxide is allowed to escape from the specimen, the pH value will shift.

CONTAINER

Capillary tube.

Syringe.

PURPOSE

To determine the pH value of the blood.

The pH value of the blood gauges the amount of free hydrogen ions that are circulating in the blood.
- pH 1–7 = acid
- pH 7–14 = alkaline.

Hydrogen is a positively charged ion. The body works to keep electrical balance between its positively charged ions, e.g. hydrogen and sodium, and the negatively charged ions, e.g. chloride and bicarbonate.

When excessive quantities of hydrogen ions are being produced, or if they become depleted, the balance of the other ions will be disturbed as they attempt to maintain electrical stability.

It is important that the body pH is kept stable.

Cell function depends on the action of enzymes, and they function most effectively at the normal pH value. Slight changes in pH will alter the speed of the reactions and disturb the physiological balance of the body.

Hydrogen ion (pH) balance is sustained through the action of the lungs and the kidneys.

Carbon dioxide is an initiator of hydrogen ion production. Increased respiratory rate and depth will remove carbon dioxide from the body and additional hydrogen ion formation is prevented.

When respiratory efforts fail to keep hydrogen ions in their correct proportions, the kidneys will excrete or conserve hydrogen ions to try and redress the balance.

Disturbances of pH balance are classified according to the system at the source of the problem.

Respiratory acidosis or respiratory alkalosis – lungs.

Metabolic acidosis or metabolic alkalosis – kidneys or increased circulating acidic products of cell metabolism, i.e. ketones.

NORMAL PHYSIOLOGY

pH is measured according to the concentration of hydrogen ions (H ions) in the body.
Raised amounts of H ions ⟶ the body becomes too acidic ⟶ lowers the pH (1–7).
Reduced amounts of H ions ⟶ the body becomes too alkaline ⟶ raises the pH (7–14).

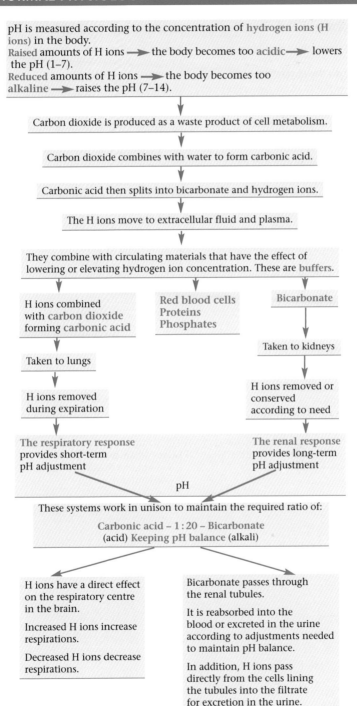

Carbon dioxide is produced as a waste product of cell metabolism.

Carbon dioxide combines with water to form carbonic acid.

Carbonic acid then splits into bicarbonate and hydrogen ions.

The H ions move to extracellular fluid and plasma.

They combine with circulating materials that have the effect of lowering or elevating hydrogen ion concentration. These are buffers.

H ions combined with carbon dioxide forming carbonic acid

Red blood cells
Proteins
Phosphates

Bicarbonate

Taken to lungs

Taken to kidneys

H ions removed during expiration

H ions removed or conserved according to need

The respiratory response provides short-term pH adjustment

The renal response provides long-term pH adjustment

pH

These systems work in unison to maintain the required ratio of:

Carbonic acid – 1 : 20 – Bicarbonate
(acid) Keeping pH balance (alkali)

H ions have a direct effect on the respiratory centre in the brain.

Increased H ions increase respirations.

Decreased H ions decrease respirations.

Bicarbonate passes through the renal tubules.

It is reabsorbed into the blood or excreted in the urine according to adjustments needed to maintain pH balance.

In addition, H ions pass directly from the cells lining the tubules into the filtrate for excretion in the urine.

ALTERED VALUES

RESPIRATORY ACIDOSIS

Retention of carbon dioxide

– Damage to the respiratory centre
  e.g. Head injury
– Obstruction of the air passages
– Reduced areas for gaseous
  exchange e.g. Emphysema
– Neuromuscular failure
  e.g. Myasthenia gravis

RESPIRATORY ALKALOSIS

Excessive elimination of carbon
dioxide
– Increased respirations
  Meningitis
  Hysterical overbreathing
  Anxiety
  Fever
  Exercise
  High altitude

METABOLIC ACIDOSIS

Excessive loss of alkali
– Diarrhoea

Failure of the kidneys to excrete
H ions
– Failure of nephron e.g. Acute
  and chronic renal failure
  Tubular acidosis
– Reduced glomerular filtrate
  Congestive cardiac failure

Accumulation of other acids
– Diabetic ketoacidosis
– Build-up of lactic acid
  Cardiac arrest
  Hypoxia
  Shock
  Exercise

METABOLIC ALKALOSIS

Excessive loss of acid
– Vomiting
– Nasogastric suction

Loss of potassium or chloride
through the kidneys
– Diuretic therapy
– Hyperaldosteronism

Cushing's disease

Effect of drugs, e.g.
– Sodium bicarbonate
– Corticosteroids

CARBON DIOXIDE/ pH BALANCE

ASSOCIATED INVESTIGATIONS

		Related pages
Carbon dioxide values	A raised blood carbon dioxide concentration will lower the blood pH.	**147**
pH	Important to measure when blood tests record an altered carbon dioxide concentration.	**150**
Oxygen values	Reflects adequacy of respiratory function.	**139**
Respirations	Altered respirations cause abnormal blood carbon dioxide concentrations. This is a cause and an effect of a raised and lowered blood pH.	**129**
Electrolyte balances		
▨ Bicarbonate	Bicarbonate values change to keep a 20:1 ratio with carbonic acid. This maintains a normal pH balance.	
▨ Potassium	Potassium moves out from its normal intracellular position to compensate for the entry of hydrogen into cells. Cells buffer the free hydrogen ions.	**102**
▨ Sodium	Attempt to provide intracellular and extracellular	**97**
▨ Chloride	electrical balance against the movement of other electrolytes.	**107**
The anion gap	Measurement of the other negative ions that make up the difference between the number of positive ions (cations) and negative ions (anions). These include magnesium, phosphates and negatively charged proteins.	
Calcium	Alkalosis can cause calcium to be lost in the urine.	**112**
Lung function tests	Investigates reasons for inadequate ventilation and the retention of carbon dioxide in the blood.	**138**
Renal function tests	Investigates reasons for the inadequate or excessive removal of hydrogen ions through the kidney.	

CONSIDERATIONS FOR CARE

RAISED BLOOD CARBON DIOXIDE VALUES

The acidotic state, a lowered pH

The basis of care lies in the treatment of the underlying disorder and the correction of the acidotic state.

The imbalance in metabolism will eventually interfere with the contractions of the cardiac muscle.

Cardiac monitoring will show dysrhythmias when they occur.

Regular measurement of the pulse and blood pressure will monitor the ability of the heart to provide an adequate circulation of blood to the tissues.

An accurate fluid balance chart will show whether an adequate cardiac output is being maintained.

If the condition continues to deteriorate, the outcome will be confusion, unconsciousness and death.

LOWERED BLOOD CARBON DIOXIDE VALUES

The state of alkalosis, a raised pH

As with acidosis, the basis of the care lies in the treatment of the underlying disorder and the correction of the state of alkalosis.

This condition causes calcium to be lost through the kidneys. The effects of alkalosis on the body are mainly due to the lowered blood calcium levels.

The hyperexcitable effect this decrease in calcium has on the nervous system will cause tetany in the muscles. Feeding and movement will become very difficult for the patient to accomplish without help.

Tetany of the respiratory muscles will lead to hypoventilation and, in severe states, respiratory arrest. Artificial ventilation may be needed to maintain life.

REFERENCE RANGE

22–26 mmol/l

PROCEDURE

Measurement from arterial blood:
- Arterial stab
- Arterial cannulation.

Apply pressure to the puncture site for at least 5 min to prevent further bleeding or bruising.

The specimen must not be exposed to air.

The specimen must be analysed immediately.

CONTAINER

Capillary tube.

Syringe.

PURPOSE

To determine the bicarbonate (HCO_3) value of the blood.

Bicarbonate (hydrogen carbonate) is derived from the sequence of changes undergone by carbon dioxide as it travels between the cell and the lungs, for expulsion during expiration. Carbon dioxide is produced as a result of adenosine triphosphate (ATP) production in the mitochondria of the cells. As carbon dioxide travels from the cells to tissues to blood it mixes with water and changes its nature.

This sequence of changes can be charted by the equation:

carbon + water $\longleftrightarrow$ carbonic acid $\longleftrightarrow$ hydrogen + bicarbonate
dioxide ions

$$CO_2 + H_2O \longleftrightarrow H_2CO_3 \longleftrightarrow H^+ + HCO_3$$

The acid–base pH balance of the body remains within its normal range when the carbonic acid and bicarbonate content of the blood is maintained in a 1:20 ratio.

As the lungs regulate carbon dioxide expulsion, it is the kidneys that remove or conserve bicarbonate according to the ratio it is holding with hydrogen ions, and the pH of the blood. If the body is becoming too acid (acidaemia), the nephrons of the kidney will conserve bicarbonate as well as excreting some hydrogen ions. If the body is becoming too alkaline (alkalaemia), the kidney nephrons will excrete surplus bicarbonate in the urine; they will also conserve hydrogen ions.

If the kidneys are unable to expel bicarbonate and an excess of bicarbonate is not maintaining the 1:20 ratio with carbonic acid, it is termed a metabolic alkalosis.

If the kidneys expel excessive amounts of bicarbonate and depletion of bicarbonate is not maintaining the 1:20 ratio with carbonic acid, it is termed a metabolic acidosis.

ALTERED VALUES

RAISED VALUES	LOWERED VALUES
Overtreatment of acidosis	Diarrhoea
Renal failure, anuria	Renal failure, unable to conserve bicarbonate

Vomiting is the expulsion of stomach contents through the mouth and nose.

Vomiting can have a basis in physical and psychological disorders, and has many causes.

It is a common symptom, frequently seen, so it is important to know when it has become a sign of disease.

Persistent vomiting can cause dehydration and electrolyte imbalance.

The consequences of this are serious for a healthy adult but are life-threatening when they apply to an infant, child or to the frail elderly.

When vomiting becomes part of a disorder, it can be the most exhausting and distressing part of the condition.

The observation of the characteristics of vomit give clues to its cause.

Many signs and symptoms are associated with vomiting:
- The feeling of nausea, salivation and retching that usually precedes vomiting can be debilitating; vomiting often relieves these symptoms.
- Heartburn caused by a reflux of stomach contents into the oesophagus gives a burning sensation. Bending over or lying down may aggravate the pain.
- Dyspepsia or indigestion, a feeling of fullness and abdominal tenderness felt after eating.
- Flatulence or 'wind' may cause discomfort and embarrassment.
- Hiccups or hiccoughs, intermittent involuntary noises made as the diaphragm contracts and pushes air through a closed glottis.

NORMAL PHYSIOLOGY

Food and drink is taken in by mouth.
Hunger, thirst and appetite influence the amount of food and drink taken.

It is cut and ground by the teeth, to form a soft bolus of food for swallowing.

Saliva is mixed with the food to:
– Moisten the food to make swallowing easier
– Add the enzyme salivary amylase; this begins the digestion of carbohydrates
– Make a fluid solution of foods and saliva, to give the sensation of taste when it makes contact with the taste buds in the mouth
– Clean the mouth after the food has been swallowed.

The food is swallowed and passes into the oesophagus.

Muscular waves or peristalsis push the food down the oesophagus. Peristalsis propels food along with alternating waves of muscular contraction and relaxation.

The gastro-oesophageal sphincter (the cardiac sphincter) is a muscular valve that separates the oesophagus from the stomach.
A wave of peristaltic relaxation goes ahead of each bolus to allow the valve to open and the food enters the stomach.

The food will remain in the stomach for several hours.

Strong muscular contractions will churn the food and mix it with gastric juice.

Gastric juice is a mixture of:
– Hydrochloric acid
– Pepsin, an enzyme that begins the process of protein digestion by making the first breaks in the amino acids chains
– Enterogastrone, the agent that prevents the stomach emptying too quickly
– The intrinsic factor, needed for the production of red blood cells
– Rennin, present in babies and young children, for digestion of milk.

The product in the stomach will now be termed 'chyme'.

The chyme will leave the stomach a little at a time through the pyloric sphincter, a muscular valve that separates the stomach from the duodenum.

The food will continue, by the action of peristalsis, to pass along the small intestine. The action of the stomach on the food will have prepared it for further breakdown by enzymes and for the products of digestion to be absorbed into the blood circulation.

THE PHYSIOLOGY OF VOMITING

The stimulation of the **vomiting centre in the medulla** of the brain.
The stimuli can be physical, psychological or emotional.

Stimulation of the vomiting centre may produce the feeling of nausea.

Nerve impulses initiate waves of **antiperistalsis** to travel up from the small intestine.

Distention of the stomach causes the vomiting to begin with strong antiperistaltic contractions of the stomach and duodenum.

The **gastrointestinal sphincter of the stomach relaxes.**

Abdominal muscles contract, pushing the stomach contents into the oesophagus.

Diaphragm contracts, abdominal muscles contract, the stomach is squeezed.

Food enters the oesophagus.

Vomitus is expelled through the mouth.

In addition to the lost food, gastric juice is also lost.
Substances expelled in vomit will include:
- Water
- Hydrogen ions
- Chloride ions
- Digestive enzymes.

OBSERVABLE CHARACTERISTICS

Force of expulsion

Vomit that has controlled force	The 'force' applies to the vomit leaving the mouth, not the strong muscular contractions that eject the vomit from the stomach. These may feel very painful and forceful.
Projectile vomiting	The vomit comes from the mouth under great force and pressure; it is propelled across the room. ■ Pyloric stenosis ■ Raised intracranial pressure.

Duration and frequency of vomit

Persistent vomiting	Vomiting that is frequent and continuous.
In relation to food	Vomiting may occur: ■ At the smell or sight of food ■ Before or after a meal ■ At a set time span after a meal ■ Caused by specific foods.
Frequency	How often the vomiting is occurring. The emergence of a pattern of vomiting.
Time of day	If the vomiting occurs at the same time each day.
Cyclical vomiting	Repeated bouts of vomiting, without a discovered cause.

Appearance of the vomit

■ Green	Gastric juice – the normal contents of the empty stomach.
■ Yellow	Bile – antiperistaltic action has brought the vomitus up from the small intestine. Bile that is secreted into the duodenum is carried along with it.
■ Red	Fresh blood – the amount of fresh blood present in the vomitus must be measured or estimated as accurately as possible. There may be flecks of fresh blood or it may be present in volume.
■ Brown	Changed blood – blood that has been in the stomach for some time and has been changed by the action of gastric secretions or Faeculent vomit – vomit that contains faecal matter. This can be due to an intestinal obstruction in the lower intestine or a fistula between the stomach and transverse colon.
■ Brown 'coffee grounds'	Changed or digested blood in the vomit, which has a granular appearance.
■ Mucus	The swallowing of excessive amounts of nasopharyngeal secretions. The vomit may appear frothy.
■ Digested food	Note the time elapsed after the meal and the amount and condition of the food.

Observable characteristics

■ Curds | Note the amount of digested milk and the time that has elapsed following a baby's milk feed.
■ Undigested food | Note the length of time passed since the food had been eaten.

■ Curds	Note the amount of digested milk and the time that has elapsed following a baby's milk feed.
■ Undigested food	Note the length of time passed since the food had been eaten.

Smell

Faecal-smelling vomit	Antiperistaltic action has brought gut contents back to the stomach from far down the gastrointestinal tract.

Other linking observations

Nausea	Feeling the need to vomit. This follows a stimulus to the vomiting centre in the brain. This unpleasant sensation may be accompanied by salivation (waterbrash), perspiration and pallor. Nausea may not precede vomiting when the cause has its origin in the brain.
Headache	Raised intracranial pressure will cause a headache with vomiting. Migraine headaches often produce vomiting.
Pain	The report of the patient on the type and place of the pain will be significant. It is also important to see whether vomiting relieves the pain, as may happen with a stomach ulcer.
Heartburn	The feeling of burning in the throat and oesophagus. This is an inflammation of the oesophagus due to a reflux of the highly acidic gastric juice through the gastro-oesophageal sphincter.
Weight loss	The prolonged loss of food and fluids will cause loss of weight.
Retching	The stomach is empty but the patient still has the antiperistaltic muscle contractions and feels the need to vomit.
Loss of appetite	The desire for food is lost, or the thought or sight of food becomes unpleasant.
Changes in bowel habits	It is important to note any changes in bowel movements that are occurring synonymously with the vomiting.

Behavioural changes

Eating disorders	Vomiting can be used by the patient as a control mechanism.
Reasons for the patient to be suffering stress or emotional upset	Vomiting can have a psychological basis.

REASONS FOR VOMITING

Infant feeding	Wind, swallowed air Taking feed too fast Normal regurgitation and posseting mistaken for vomiting Overfeeding Feeding intolerances Indicator of gastrointestinal disorders and other diseases.
Intestinal obstruction	Vomiting will occur when the stomach or duodenum is full and the food is unable to empty from the stomach. This may occur after each meal, or late each day as the stomach becomes more full with each meal.
Gastritis	Inflammation of the stomach mucosa. The cause may be external from ingested food or drugs or internal auto-immune conditions, i.e. pernicious anaemia.
Infection	Vomiting is not confined to direct infection of the gastrointestinal tract. Other sites of infection will cause vomiting, i.e. urinary tract infections.
With prolonged coughing attacks	When excessive amounts of mucus are swallowed. Whooping cough.
Emotion	Sights and situations that cause emotional turmoil.
Eating disorders	Vomiting as part of a psychological disorder.
Pain	Severe pain may cause nausea and vomiting.
Travel sickness	Disturbance to the inner ear and balance will cause dizziness, nausea and vomiting.
Poisoning	e.g. Alcohol.
Drugs	Emetics, cytotoxic therapy, opiates.
Raised intracranial pressure	Vomiting following a head injury is a serious sign. It is one of the signs of a raised intracranial pressure.
Pregnancy	Morning sickness.
General anaesthesia	The stomach must be empty at the time of anaesthetic. If vomiting occurs while the patient is without a cough reflex, stomach contents can enter the air passages.
Metabolic disorders	Ketoacidosis, uraemia.

ASSOCIATED INVESTIGATIONS

		Related pages
pH	The loss of hydrogen ions with the gastric juice will eventually cause an alkalosis. Sugar and carbohydrate foods continually lost from the stomach will initiate the breakdown of stored fats for energy and the development of ketoacidosis.	150
Electrolyte values		
▦ Chloride	Chloride values will be lowered when hydrochloric acid is lost from the stomach.	107
▦ Potassium	Potassium will not be absorbed by the gastrointestinal tract; values will therefore fall.	102
▦ Sodium	Sodium will not be absorbed by the gastrointestinal tract; values will therefore fall.	97
Abdominal X-ray	The pictures are able to show evidence of obstruction in the gastrointestinal tract.	295
A fluid intake and output chart	The fluid intake side of the chart will record: ▦ The oral fluid (and food) intake or attempted intake ▦ The fluid input through an intravenous infusion The fluid output side of the chart will record: ▦ The number of episodes, amount and description of vomit ▦ The urinary output: a diminished urinary output, when renal disease is not the basic problem, may signify dehydration.	
Signs of dehydration	Loss of skin elasticity. Dry mucous membranes, sunken eyes, poor urine output. A baby will have depressed fontanelles.	
Temperature	A rise in temperature may indicate that an infection is the cause of the vomiting.	4
Pulse Blood pressure	These vital signs will alter if dehydration is causing a strain on the cardiovascular system. Raised intracranial pressure as a cause of vomiting will slow the pulse and the blood pressure will rise.	9 17
Endoscopy	Direct imaging of the gastrointestinal tract.	

CONSIDERATIONS FOR CARE

Vomiting is a distressing matter for most people. They find it embarrassing and stressful.

If it is known that the person may vomit, a bowl and tissues must be made ready in a discreet but accessible place to save the patient all possible anxiety should the event occur.

If vomiting does happen, privacy and help must be given while the episode persists.

Once the patient feels a little better, give them a mouth wash. Change clothing and linen that has been marked by the vomitus.

The person may feel uneasy about needing help with these unpleasant tasks, and it will be up to the carer to create an atmosphere where the patient's dignity remains intact.

Each vomit should be recorded.

The time, the amount and the characteristics of the vomit should be noted.

If an unconscious or anaesthetised patient vomits, they must be correctly positioned on their side to avoid choking. Suction must be available for use.

If the vomiting persists, signs of dehydration must be watched for. An intravenous infusion may be needed to compensate for the loss of oral fluids and electrolytes.

When it is thought that food and fluids could be tolerated, they must be offered in small amounts, with a gradual build-up to a normal diet.

If vomiting persists, keep a record of weight loss.

Anti-emetics and antacids are helpful medications for the control of vomiting.

Local laboratory specifications will need to be followed when stool samples are taken for testing. The potentially contagious nature of a stool means that strict precautions must be taken when dealing with these specimens.

Taking a specimen of stool for laboratory testing:
- Wear gloves when using the spatula to transfer the stool specimen to the specimen pot
- The stool specimen should be collected from a contaminant-free container
- The specimen should not be allowed to dry out
- If the specimen cannot be tested immediately, it may be kept in a refrigerator.

3- or 5-day stool collection:
- The collecting pot should be labelled with the start and finish date and time
- Bowel preparations should not be used during the time that the stools are collected.

The application of normal measurements that are applied to the excretion of faeces can only be used to refer uniquely to one individual, and the pattern of bowel habits that they are accustomed to. The term 'normal' then becomes very wide ranging.

Abnormalities become variations on long-standing patterns of faecal excretion.

Changes may occur in:
- The colour of the stool
- The consistency of the stool
- The frequency that stools are passed
- Presence of offensive odour
- Blood may become apparent when the bowels are opened
- Pain when defaecating
- The ability to remain continent of faeces.

INFANTS

Expected changes in the colour and consistency of stools will occur during the first week of life:
- Meconium   The first stool of the newborn.
                   The stool is black and tarry. It has no odour.
- Changing stool   Occurs about the third day of life.
                   The stool becomes green.
- Baby stool   From the fifth day of life.
                   The stool will be yellow and formed:
                   - Pale yellow if breast fed
                   - Dark yellow if bottle fed.

NORMAL PHYSIOLOGY

Chyme from the stomach enters the duodenum.

The small intestine absorbs:
■ Amino acids as the breakdown products of proteins
■ Sugars as the breakdown products of carbohydrates
■ Chylomicrons or droplets of fat.

The remaining substances pass through the ileocaecal valve into the large intestine.

Chyme passing through the large intestine will contain:
■ Water   ■ Epithelial cells
■ Undigested foods   ■ Bacteria
■ Cellulose   ■ Mucus
■ Salts   ■ Colouring from the bile pigments,
                               stercobilin and urobilin

Peristalsis squeezes and turns the **chyme, moving it slowly along the length of the colon.**

The walls of the colon:
■ Absorb water
■ Absorb sodium and chloride
■ Secrete a mucus containing sodium bicarbonate. This protects the walls of the colon from the action of bacteria, and the acidic end products of digestion.

Colonic bacteria:
■ Produce vitamin K
■ Digest some cellulose.

As the chyme moves slowly through the colon, it changes from a liquid to a solid state.

Faecal matter gradually builds up in the rectum.

Faecal incontinence is prevented by two valves, an internal and an external sphincter muscle.

The anatomical bend at the end of the colon also controls the passage of faeces.

When the rectum reaches a point of distension, the urge to defaecate is produced.

This reaction is also produced by the gastrointestinal reflex, initiated when food enters the stomach.

The stimulus to evacuate the bowel is under conscious control. If circumstances for defaecation are not correct, the urge to empty the rectum will stop.

A stool will be passed when:
■ The nervous impulses produce waves of peristalsis in the colon and rectum
■ The diaphragm is fixed and the breath is held
■ The abdominal muscles contract, pushing the faeces down the rectum
■ The external sphincter opens
■ The pelvic floor muscles stretch and the anus opens.

ABNORMAL STOOLS

A CHANGE IN COLOUR

The normal brown stool colour is due to bile pigments and the breakdown products of red blood cells.

Food dyes may produce a change of colour, e.g. beetroot.

Pale clay colour	Obstructive biliary disease preventing the secretion of bile into the duodenum.
Grey	High fat content in stool.
Green	Rapid passage through the intestine does not allow the chyme to change colour. In babies: ■ Hunger ■ Overfeeding.
Black	Digested blood in the stool. Melaena, may have a tarry consistency. ■ Bleeding into the upper gastrointestinal tract ■ Swallowed blood.
Bright red	Frank fresh blood in or on the stool. The stool may only be flecked with blood. Bleeding into the lower bowel or at the anus.
White	Remains of barium from an investigation.

A CHANGE IN CONSISTENCY

A formed stool usually takes the shape of the rectum, where it has been stored.

Fluid stool	Diarrhoea. ■ The transit of chyme through the colon is too rapid for sufficient water to be absorbed to form a stool ■ The food substances that are bulking materials in the formation of stools have not been eaten ■ Liquid faecal material, with the appearance of diarrhoea, will leak around faeces that have become impacted in the rectum and colon.
Liquid stool with a seedy appearance	In babies, rapid transit of chyme through the gastrointestina tract, with the undigested milk curds giving the seedy look to the stool.
Hard solid stools	Constipation. The stool has been stored in the rectum for a long time and water has continued to be absorbed from the stool.
Stringy or ribbon shaped	An obstruction has changed the shape of the stools in the rectum.
Bulky Frothy Greasy	Malabsorptive disease, affecting the absorption of fat. These stools have an offensive odour. They float in the toilet.
Redcurrent jelly stool	The name describes the look of the stool. In babies, an indication of intussusception.

Abnormal stools

INABILITY TO DEFAECATE

No passage of stools from the rectum:
- The rectum may be impacted with faeces and be unable to evacuate
- An obstruction is preventing the rectum filling with faeces
- An abnormality of the muscles or the nerve supply to the gut is preventing the passage of chyme along the gastrointestinal tract.

PAINFUL DEFAECATION

Abdominal pain:
- Colonic contractions that accompany defaecation will be painful when the bowel is inflamed.

Muscular pain:
- Injury or surgery to the abdominal muscles will cause pain when these muscles are contracted for defaecation.

Perineal and anal pain:
- Injury or surgery to the perineal muscles will cause pain when they stretch to allow defaecation
- Local conditions of the anus, e.g. haemorrhoids and anal fissures, will cause great discomfort when the anus needs to stretch.

REASONS FOR ALTERED STOOLS

DIARRHOEA

Irritation of the colon wall causing increased peristalsis	Increased peristalsis increases the rate of chyme movement through the gastrointestinal tract. Causes are: ■ Pathogenic organisms ■ Food sensitivity ■ Inflammation of the bowel.
Destruction of intestinal mucosa	Water and salt absorption from the colon is prevented. Causes are: ■ Pathogenic organisms ■ Inflammation.
Inability to absorb specific nutrients (malabsorption)	Nutrients pass undigested through the gut taking a large volume of fluid with them.
Conditions that increase gastrointestinal mobility	■ Raised metabolic rate, e.g. thyrotoxicosis ■ Diabetic autonomic neuropathy ■ Following gastric surgery.
Physiological reaction to psychological stress	Stress causes increased nervous activity to the bowel, increasing gut motility.
Irritable bowel syndrome	The diarrhoea may be attributed to physiological or psychological causes.
Overuse of laxatives	
Reaction to antibiotic therapy	

CONSTIPATED STOOLS

Slow movement of chyme through the colon	An increased amount of water is absorbed from the stool. It becomes hard and dry. Causes include: ■ Immobility ■ Hypothyroidism.
Inadequate roughage in diet Inadequate fluid intake	Insufficient bulking material or water in the formed stool.
Weak colonic muscles to push through and evacuate waste	Difficult transit of faeces for excretion. Causes include: ■ Long-term use of laxatives ■ Colonic spasm.
Holding the stool in the rectum for a long period of time	When the feeling of need to defaecate is ignored, it will subside. If the feeling is always ignored it will stop completely. Causes include: ■ Painful defaecation ■ Unsuitable environment ■ Incorrect toilet training.
Obstruction to the passage of faeces in the colon	■ New growths ■ Torsion ■ Inflammation and oedema.

Reasons for altered stools

Dysfunctional nervous system supplying large bowel	Paralytic ileus. The gut reacts to being handled during surgery. Spinal injury: ■ The loss of sensation for the need to pass a stool ■ The inability to push out the stool. The absence of nervous tissue in part of the bowel – Hirschsprung's disease.
Drugs	Including: ■ Codeine ■ Opiates.

STEATORRHOEA

Stools that have a high fat content.

They appear pale in colour, and are bulky and frothy, with an offensive odour. They float in a toilet.

Bile not available to break down ingested fat particles	■ Liver disease prevents the manufacture of bile. ■ Bile ducts between liver, gall bladder and duodenum are blocked. Causes are: 　■ Inflammation 　■ Stones 　■ New growths.
Pancreatic lipase not available to break down fats into fatty acids and monoglycerides	Diseased pancreas unable to manufacture pancreatic juice or its components.
Small intestine unable to absorb the products of fat digestion	■ Non-functioning or absence of villi on wall of small intestine. ■ Surgical removal of portion of small intestine.

MELAENA

The stool is black in colour and may be 'tarry' in consistency. The stool contains blood that has entered high up in the gastrointestinal tract and the blood has been through the digestive processes.

As the bleeding point is in the upper part of the gut, the patient may also be vomiting coffee grounds or flesh blood. Causes:
■ Erosion of the gastrointestinal mucosa
■ Bleeding varices
■ New growths
■ Haemorrhagic disease
■ Swallowed blood from injury or post-operative bleeding.

ASSOCIATED INVESTIGATIONS

		Related pages
Stool chart	To keep a record of the time and type of stools that are passed.	150
Fluid input and output chart	To ensure sufficient fluids are given: ■ To replace fluid lost by diarrhoea ■ To prevent constipation.	
Electrolyte levels	The large bowel absorbs sodium and chloride and secretes bicarbonate.	97 107
Culture and sensitivity	To isolate pathogens that are causing diarrhoea and to select the antibiotic for treatment, if appropriate.	294
Microscopic investigation for parasites	Stool examined for parasitic organisms or their eggs.	
Test for occult blood	The presence of blood may not be obvious in the stool. Many foods give a false-positive result.	
Faecal urobilinogen	Urobilin, the bile pigment, gives stools their brown colour. Decreased content indicates that bile is not reaching the chyme, through liver disease or obstruction of the biliary tract.	
Tests for malabsorption	■ Xylose tolerance test – to determine the ability of the small intestine to absorb complex sugars ■ Faecal fat ■ Reducing substances ■ Pancreatic function tests.	
Endoscopes	■ Sigmoidoscopy – examination and biopsy of the lower colon and rectum ■ Proctoscopy – examination and biopsy of the rectum ■ Colonoscopy.	
X-ray examination	Barium enema	295
Scans	■ Ultrasound examination ■ Computerised tomography.	298 296

CONSIDERATIONS FOR CARE

Open discussion about bowel habits may be perceived as socially unacceptable. The patient may feel great discomfort when they need to talk about it. This sensitivity is countered by health care staff who have generally lost all embarrassment about the subject by frequently dealing with the theme. The attitude of the listener is important to set the right conditions for the patient to feel comfortable.

The normal pattern of bowel habits should be ascertained before changes can be assessed.

This background information may be evaluated against the type of food normally included in the diet.

Having documented the normal pattern of bowel movements, the patient's diet and fluid intake may need to be adapted.

Normal bowel routine is often upset when a patient enters hospital. Communal toilets, commodes and bedpans can have an inhibiting effect. The immobility of bedrest and the unnatural position adopted when using a bedpan can constrain defaecation. Privacy is always necessary.

Communal toilets must be clean and have working locks on the door.

A patient with diarrhoea must be placed near a toilet. The toilet should remain for the use of this patient only. Handwashing facilities must be close by.

An immobile patient will need a call bell and the calls should be answered promptly.

The basis of care will be to find the cause of the condition and, if possible, treat it.

Extra fluids may be given orally or intravenously to prevent dehydration occurring.

Electrolyte balance may also need correcting.

A constipated patient will need:
■ To find the reason for the constipation
■ To find a remedy to the initial problem
■ To remove the faeces from the bowel, through medications or manual means
■ To take measures to prevent the condition reoccurring. At the simplest level, this can mean an alteration to their diet or taking more exercise.

Faecal incontinence must be dealt with competently, to help the patient keep their self-respect and comfort. If it becomes a chronic problem, skin around the sacral area will need protection.

URINE FOR TESTING

Specimens must be collected in clean containers.

The specimen should be clean, uncontaminated by faeces, penile or vaginal discharge or menstrual fluid.

Delay in testing the urine will cause alterations in the measured results.

Staff should wear protective gloves when dealing with urine specimens.

Local policies and procedures should be followed when obtaining the specimen of urine.

This especially applies to the collection of a catheter specimen when an incorrect technique will introduce infection into the urinary tract.

An early morning urine is the best specimen to test:
- Having fasted overnight, the urine test results will not be affected by the recent absorption of food components
- The substances that are sought by the urine test will be accumulating in the bladder overnight
- The lack of fluid intake overnight will concentrate the tested substances in the bladder.

The early morning urine specimen of a diabetic patient will not give accurate measurements:
- Urine that has accumulated in the bladder overnight will not reflect the blood glucose and ketone values in the early morning
- The bladder will need to be emptied, then the specimen of urine collected one hour later.

Observations made prior to testing the urine:
- The patient reports pain, or dysuria, when passing urine.
- The patient has difficulty starting the flow of urine.
- The colour of the urine should be pale to a golden yellow.

A dark coloured urine may contain:
- Red food dyes, i.e. beetroot
- Haematuria
- Bilirubin, causes marks on underwear.

A urine that turns red in the light is a sign of the condition porphyria.

Injected dyes used for investigation purposes, that are excreted through the kidney, will colour the urine.
- Frothy urine can indicate a high protein content.
- The odour of the urine should not be offensive. A 'fishy' odour will be caused by infection in the urinary tract. An ammonia smell comes from stale urine.
- The urine should be clear when held up to the light.

Threads or casts will appear when the urinary tract is inflamed or infected.

These are formed in the renal tubules, or as leucocyte casts during urinary tract infections.

URINE TESTING

ROUTINE URINALYSIS

The use of chemical and stick reagents.

Accurate testing depends on:
- Using a correct method when collecting the urine specimen
- The use of clean, rinsed containers
- An uncontaminated specimen of urine
- Following the manufacturer's instructions when using the reagents.

SUPRAPUBIC ASPIRATION

Used to obtain a sterile urine specimen from a person who is unable to co-operate with instructions to provide one, i.e. babies, incontinent or confused patients.

A full bladder is palpated. From a position just above the symphysis pubis, a sterile needle is inserted into the bladder and a specimen of urine is syringed back.

MID-STREAM SPECIMEN OF URINE

To obtain a specimen of urine free from contaminants.
- Local policy and procedure must be followed to obtain this specimen of urine.
- All areas of tissue that may come into contact with the urine specimen need to be washed free of contaminating organisms.
- The initial part of the flow of urine needs to be discarded. This will contain tissue debris from the urethra and the urinary meatus.
- The urine is then collected in a sterile container.
- Care needs to be taken that the inside of the container is not contaminated by fingers.

CATHETER SPECIMEN OF URINE

- Local policy and procedure must be followed when collecting this specimen of urine.
- The urine may not be taken from the collecting bag.
- The specimen must be fresh urine, taken in its passage down from the bladder into the collection tubing.
- The line between the catheter and the collecting bag must not be broken. This would risk introducing infection into the urinary tract.

RESIDUAL URINE

This procedure measures the amount of urine left after the bladder has been emptied voluntarily.

Local policy and procedure should be followed when introducing a catheter into the bladder for the residual urine to drain off.

24-HOUR COLLECTION OF URINE

- Local policy and procedure must be followed when this collection of urine is taken.
- Urine is passed and discarded at the time the specimen collection begins.
- If a specimen of urine is inadvertently thrown away during the 24 hours, the collection must recommence.

REFERENCE RANGE

Adult: Average output 800–2500 ml each 24 hours

Child: Varies with age, 600–1000 ml each 24 hours

Neonate: 2–4 ml/kg/hour

PROCEDURE

Measure and record each quantity of urine passed.

If incontinence prevents the measurement of urine, a system of quantifying the amount passed must be used, i.e. damp, (+), (++), (+++), (++++).

Nappies: the weight of the wet nappy should be subtracted from the nappy's dry weight, to measure the amount of urine passed (1 g = 1 ml urine).

PURPOSE

To ensure that sufficient urine is passed to eliminate the waste substances that are filtered and excreted by the kidneys.

Water circulating as part of the blood passes through the kidneys. Most of the water is reabsorbed by capillaries around the kidney tubule and put back into the circulation, but excess water passes through the kidney tubule to be excreted.

The water that passes on through the kidney has other waste products for excretion (the solutes) dissolved in it, to form urine.

There is an upper limit to the amount of solutes that can be dissolved in a given volume of water. Sufficient water must be circulated through the kidney tubules to dilute the waste products.

An excess of water compared to the amount of solutes to be concentrated will produce a dilute urine.

When a minimum amount of water is available for dilution of solutes, the urine becomes concentrated.

It is the sensation of thirst that ensures that sufficient fluids are taken to maintain a correct blood volume and provide the kidneys with adequate water in which to dissolve the solutes.

The ability of the kidneys to concentrate urine varies with age. The immature kidney of the neonate will pass frequent amounts of dilute urine. In health, kidney function will improve with maturity until in old age it again becomes less efficient. The ability to concentrate the urine recedes and more water is needed to dilute the solute load. More urine will need to be passed. Nocturia may then follow.

NORMAL PHYSIOLOGY

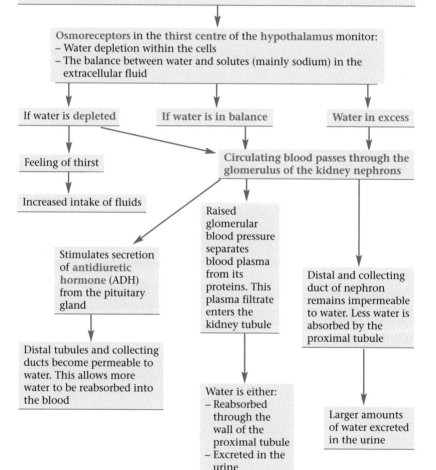

Water intake
– Oral fluids
– Water content of floods
– Metabolic breakdown of foods

99% of integested water is absorbed into the tissues through the walls of the large and small intenstine and becomes part of the:
– Plasma
– Interstitial fluid
– Intracellular fluid

Osmoreceptors in the **thirst centre** of the **hypothalamus** monitor:
– Water depletion within the cells
– The balance between water and solutes (mainly sodium) in the extracellular fluid

| If water is depleted | If water is in balance | Water in excess |

Feeling of thirst

Increased intake of fluids

Circulating blood passes through the glomerulus of the kidney nephrons

Stimulates secretion of **antidiuretic hormone** (ADH) from the pituitary gland

Distal tubules and collecting ducts become permeable to water. This allows more water to be reabsorbed into the blood

Raised glomerular blood pressure separates blood plasma from its proteins. This plasma filtrate enters the kidney tubule

Water is either:
– Reabsorbed through the wall of the proximal tubule
– Excreted in the urine

Distal and collecting duct of nephron remains impermeable to water. Less water is absorbed by the proximal tubule

Larger amounts of water excreted in the urine

ALTERED VALUES

RAISED URINE VALUES

Polyuria

Polydipsia

Increased osmotic load in urine
– Glycosuria
– High urea content

Diabetes insipidus
– Defect in production of antidiuretic hormone
– Defective renal response to antidiuretic hormone

Renal disease
Decreased ability of nephrons to concentrate urine
– Medullary cystic disease
– Potassium depletion
– Hypercalcaemia

Recovery from oedema

– No urine is passed
Effect of drugs, including:
– Diuretic drugs
– Alcohol

FREQUENCY OF MICTURITION

Differs from polyuria

A normal volume of urine is passed but it is passed in frequent small amounts

Urinary tract infections

Obstruction of the urinary pathways
– Enlarged prostate
– Presence of a blood clot

LOWERED URINE VALUES

Oliguria

Reduced fluid intake

Dehydration
– Nausea and vomiting
– Diarrhoea
– Poorly planned 'nil by mouth' regime

Overproduction of the antidiuretic hormone from the pituitary gland
– Raised sodium level

Post-operative stress

Renal disease
– Nephrotic syndrome

Poor blood flow to kidneys
– Hypotension
– Congestive cardiac failure

ANURIA

– Lack of blood supply to both kidneys
– Complete obstruction of urinary pathway from both kidneys

URINARY RETENTION

Urine in bladder but patient is unable to pass it
– Post-operative trauma
– Pain or fear of pain
– Urethral inflammation or obstruction

ASSOCIATED INVESTIGATIONS

		Related pages
Fluid input and output chart	To measure the difference in volume of fluids taken in and the amount of urine excreted. Also to ensure that sufficient fluids are taken to dilute the solute load when urine is formed.	
Routine urine analysis	To ensure that a normal solute load is being carried by the water in the urine.	174
Blood glucose	An outcome of a raised blood glucose will be glycosuria. Glucose is an osmotic diuretic. Urine volume will rise as the amount of glucose excreted by the kidneys increases.	85
Specific gravity of urine	To measure the dilution of the urine.	180
Osmolality of urine and plasma	To calculate the amount of osmotic pull exercised by the solutes carried in the urine and the blood.	
Daily weight	Rapid, excessive changes in weight can be accounted for by the accumulation or loss of body fluids.	264
The presence of oedema	A positive sign of fluid retention.	283
Blood values of ■ Sodium ■ Potassium ■ Chloride ■ Bicarbonate	The response and the ability of the kidneys to maintain homeostasis.	97 102 107
Blood values of ■ Urea ■ Creatinine	To test the ability of the kidney to excrete waste products, produced by metabolism. Urea, like glucose, is an osmotic diuretic. An increased volume of urine will accompany the passage of an increased urea concentration through the kidney.	121 119
Creatinine clearance test	To assess the function of the renal tubules by measuring their ability to excrete waste products.	
Uroflowmetry	Urine is passed through a flowmeter that assesses the volume, rate and pattern of urine flow.	

CONSIDERATIONS FOR CARE

RAISED URINE VOLUME

When the kidneys excrete excessive amounts of water, the dehydrating effect on the body stimulates the thirst centre in the hypothalamus.

If the patient can respond to this by taking oral fluids, drinks should be provided.

When oral rehydration is not possible, fluid replacement therapy by nasogastric feeding or intravenous infusion should be initiated.

An accurate fluid balance chart must be maintained to prevent excessive rehydration.

The underlying cause should, if possible, be treated.

'Frequency of urine' may give the impression that a larger than usual volume of urine is being passed, but the amounts when measured may add up to a normal volume of urine.

'Urgency to pass urine' does not give the patient much time between feeling the need to urinate and the bladder expelling the urine. The distress that this causes can be reduced by placing the patient a short distance from the toilet. When the patient is immobile, they must have access to a call bell, and requests for bedpans and commodes must be answered promptly.

Incontinence of urine, whether in children or adults, is a problem that must be dealt with carefully and tactfully. A poor attitude from the carer will further undermine the person's self-respect and create further problems.

If incontinence allows urine to make contact with the skin, excellent hygiene and skin protection will be necessary. Rapid remedial action by carers will reduce odour, skin damage and discomfort. Clean clothes and linen must be available for immediate changes when necessary.

Introducing a programme of toilet retraining to deal with a problem of incontinence in older children needs careful planning. Analysis of the causes of the problem and consideration of the individual child's situation and development must be made.

LOWERED URINE VOLUME

The cause of the decreased urine volume must be investigated.

If the cause is dehydration, additional fluids will need to be given to increase the volume of water in the blood circulation. This therapy may not be appropriate if the decrease in urine flow is due to kidney disease or obstruction in the urinary system. In these circumstances, careful control of fluid intake will be necessary to avoid further damaging effects.

If catheterisation of the bladder is used as a remedy for incontinence or retention of urine, strict adherence to local policies regarding catheter care is essential. These will help to avoid the introduction of infection into the system, damage to the neck of the bladder, and allow free flow of urine.

URINE SPECIFIC GRAVITY

NORMAL MEASUREMENT

A specific gravity between 1002 and 1025.

PROCEDURE

A specific gravity-sensitive urine test stick.

A urinometer.

PURPOSE

The specific gravity of urine indicates the quantity of dissolved substances present in the urine.

The baseline is a specific gravity of 1000. This is the specific gravity of distilled water.

As water travels through the kidney nephron, it carries with it dissolved salts, minerals and other waste products. The specific gravity will rise above 1000 according to the weight of the concentrated solutes dissolved in the water.

The specific gravity will rise with the increasing molecular weight of the particles within the water.

The work of the kidney nephrons is to:
- Take waste products from the plasma and excrete them
- Maintain homeostasis by reabsorption of substances when deficiencies occur, or by excretion when excesses occur.

When a substance enters the nephron, it is reabsorbed back into the blood circulation or excreted in the urine according to the body's need. To re-enter the circulation, some substances will need a method of transport across the wall of the nephron. When the substance is in excess, all means of transport will become exhausted. This indicates that the renal threshold has been reached and that substance will pass along the nephron and appear in the urine. A rise in urine specific gravity will then be seen, especially if the substance has a high molecular weight, such as glucose.

Specific gravity readings and urine output should be considered concurrently.

When nephrons lose their capacity to alter the filtrate, the urine becomes nearer the specific gravity of the filtrate taken from the blood at the glomerulus.

When kidney nephrons no longer function:

Urine specific gravity = glomerular filtrate specific gravity = 1008

This becomes a fixed specific gravity value; isosthenuria.

ALTERED VALUES

RAISED VALUES

Reduced volume of urinary water
– Dehydration
– Oedema
– Diarrhoea

Raised urea content in urine
– Dehydration

Raised glucose content in urine
– Diabetes mellitus

Osmotic diuretics
– Increased urea values
– Increased glucose values
– Mannitol
Urine volume is also increased.

LOWERED VALUES

Increased volume of urinary water
– Overhydration
– Kidney dysfunction, causing an
  inability to concentrate urine
– Diabetes insipidus

Decreased sodium content
– Salt-restricted diets

Decreased urea content in urine
– Low protein diet

ASSOCIATED INVESTIGATIONS

Related pages

Fluid input and output chart	Will indicate a lack of balance between urinary output and: ■ The amount of fluid taken in ■ The amount of urine needed to excrete the solute load.	
Routine urinalysis	Tests for the presence of abnormal constituents in the urine and solutes in excessive amounts. This will raise the urine specific gravity.	**174**
Colour of the urine	A concentrated urine with a high specific gravity will be darker in colour. A dilute urine with a low specific gravity will be pale in colour.	
Plasma and urine osmolality	To compare and ensure that the solute content of the urine and plasma are within normal limits, and in the correct dilution. Solutes attract water with an osmotic pull. By calculating the combined solute pull in a given weight of water and comparing it with the amount of water present, the dilution of the urine and plasma can be calculated, and the ability of the kidney to concentrate urine.	
Water deprivation test	To test the ability of the kidneys to concentrate urine.	
Pulse and blood pressure	Overhydration and dehydration will affect the circulatory volume. Changes in blood volume will be reflected in pulse and blood pressure measurements.	**9** **17**

CONSIDERATIONS FOR CARE

RAISED SPECIFIC GRAVITY

A raised specific gravity means that the solute content of the urine is high.

Investigations must decide whether the increase is caused by:
- An increased solute content in the normal volume of urine or
- A normal solute content in a decreased volume of urine.

An increased solute load that has diuretic properties, e.g. glucose or urea, will increase the specific gravity and the urine volume.

Care and treatment will depend on identifying the solute causing the rise in specific gravity and finding the cause for this imbalance.

If specific gravity has risen because of a lack of water in the urine, the cause may lie either in:
- A reduced fluid intake or
- Fluid retention in the tissues of the body.

The distinction must be made before a fluid replacement therapy is begun.

To initiate fluid replacement therapy when the kidneys are unable to maintain fluid homeostasis will cause circulatory volume overload.

Fluid retention in the tissues may be apparent as oedema. If oedema is present, particular precautions must be taken to protect the areas of swollen skin, especially where there is pressure or a risk of wounding.

The high fluid content of oedematous tissues and the circulatory stasis will make healing a difficult process.

LOW SPECIFIC GRAVITY

A low specific gravity means that the solute content of the urine is low.

Investigations must decide whether the decrease is caused by:
- A decreased solute content in a normal volume of urine or
- A normal solute content in an increased volume of water.

Unless there is a specific reason to withhold fluids, drinks should be encouraged as they are beneficial to all aspects of health.

When the mechanisms controlling the excretion of water are damaged, the water content of the urine will increase and the solute levels will fall. This is seen dramatically when the production of antidiuretic hormone ceases.

Fluid replacement therapy and treatment of the underlying cause will be needed to maintain life.

URINE pH

REFERENCE RANGE

Normal pH value 4.3–8.

PROCEDURE

Urine pH reagent stick.

Testing should be on fresh urine, as urine left to stand will become alkaline.

PURPOSE

pH measures the hydrogen ion concentration in the urine.

To function properly, the cells of the body need to be maintained at pH 7.4.

The control mechanisms that keep the pH constant lie with the lungs and the kidneys.

To keep the pH balance:
- Lungs alter the rate at which carbon dioxide is expelled from the body
- Kidneys conserve or excrete bicarbonate according to the body's need. They also excrete excess free hydrogen ions from the circulation. It is the quantity of free hydrogen ions in the urine that gives the pH value.

When the lungs are unable to rid the body of sufficient carbon dioxide, an excess of free H^+ ions are in circulation – a state of respiratory acidosis.

To counter this and keep the body in balance the kidneys will:
- Conserve bicarbonate and maintain its ratio of 1:20 with carbonic acid
- Excrete more hydrogen ions in the urine.

The urine pH will fall; it will become more acid.

When the lungs rid the body of too much carbon dioxide, unbuffered hydrogen ions to be excreted by the kidney will be reduced. This reduction of hydrogen ions will cause the urine to become more alkaline and the pH will rise.

The pH value of urine will also be affected by the acidity and alkalinity of other solutes dissolved in the urine.

NORMAL PHYSIOLOGY

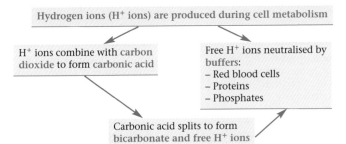

Hydrogen ions (H^+ ions) are produced during cell metabolism

H^+ ions combine with carbon dioxide to form carbonic acid

Free H^+ ions neutralised by buffers:
– Red blood cells
– Proteins
– Phosphates

Carbonic acid splits to form bicarbonate and free H^+ ions

The acid–base (pH) balance of the body is maintained when the quantities of circulating carbonic acid (acid) and bicarbonate (alkali/base) are kept in a 1 : 20 ratio

Carbonic acid values regulated by the lungs

Bicarbonate values regulated by the kidneys

Bicarbonate enters the kidney nephron with the filtrate

It combines with free H^+ ions to re-form into carbonic acid

The carbonic acid splits into carbon dioxide and water

The carbon dioxide is reabsorbed into the blood circulation where it combines with water again to make more bicarbonate

This chain of events adjusts to manufacture or excrete more bicarbonate through the kidneys to maintain the carbonic acid : bicarbonate ratio at 1 : 20, and keep the body pH at 7.4

In addition:

Free circulating H^+ ions are excreted by the kidney to maintain a body pH of 7.4.

They enter the renal filtrate from the cells surrounding the lumen of the kidney tubule.

The H^+ ions are buffered in the urine by:

– Phosphates
– Ammonia.

When the body excretes an excess of H^+ ions exceeding the buffering capacity, free H^+ ions will appear in the urine and the pH of the urine will fall (become more acidic).

When the body is conserving H^+ ions and the buffering capacity is adequate, fewer free H^+ ions will appear in the urine and the pH of the urine will rise (become more alkaline).

ACID/ALKALINE VALUES

ACID	ALKALINE	
pH 1–7	Neutral	pH 7–14
Respiratory acidosis caused by: Retention of carbon dioxide. – Disorders of respiration preventing adequate expiration		Respiratory alkalosis caused by: Excess expiration of carbon dioxide. – Disorders of respiration causing hyperventilation
Metabolic acidosis – Diabetes mellitus – Starvation		Metabolic alkalosis
		Renal tubular acidosis Reduced excretion of H^+ ions caused by defects of renal tubules
Loss of alkali – Diarrhoea		Loss of acid – Vomiting
Diet high in meat		Diet high in fruit and vegetables
		Urinary tract infection with ammonia-producing bacteria
Effects of drugs, including: – Ascorbic acid		Effect of drugs, including: – Sodium bicarbonate – Potassium citrate – Sodium citrate

ASSOCIATED INVESTIGATIONS

Related pages

Blood pH	To see if the abnormal urine pH reflects an abnormal blood pH.	
Blood carbon dioxide	The retention of carbon dioxide in the blood will cause the kidney to excrete hydrogen ions. This will lower the urine pH.	147
Blood bicarbonate values	The retention of carbon dioxide in the blood will cause the kidneys to conserve bicarbonate. This balance between bicarbonate and carbonic acid levels keeps blood pH stable.	
Blood oxygen values	Indicates the adequacy of respiratory function and reflects the ability of the body to eliminate carbon dioxide.	139
Lung function tests	To investigate the inability of the lungs to eliminate carbon dioxide from the body.	138
Renal function tests	To investigate the inability of the kidney to excrete or conserve hydrogen ions or bicarbonate in the proper proportions.	
Urine test for culture and sensitivity	To detect the presence of bacteria that can cause urine to become abnormally alkaline.	294
Blood glucose Urine glucose Urinary ketones	When glucose cannot be used as an energy source for cell metabolism, fats and proteins can be converted to replace glucose. When this happens, ketone bodies form and are excreted in the urine. They are acidic and lower urine pH.	85 193
Urinary ketones	The presence of ketones lowers the pH of the urine.	197

CONSIDERATIONS FOR CARE

A RAISED URINE pH

Alkaline urine

The basis of care depends on the cause of the abnormally alkaline urine.

Unassisted prolonged hyperventilation is physically difficult to maintain. Hyperventilation may be associated with a prolonged set expiratory time when a patient is requiring mechanical ventilation.

A metabolic alkalosis will be caused by the loss of acid from the body through vomiting or through the kidneys.

Treatment of the causative condition and correction of the electrolyte loss by intravenous or oral means is required.

A LOWERED URINE pH

Acid urine

Care given will depend on the cause of the abnormally acid urine.

If respiratory impairment prevents the elimination of carbon dioxide from the body, steps need to be taken to improve lung function:
- Positioning the patient to allow maximum lung expansion
- Giving medications to improve lung efficiency
- Oxygen therapy, if appropriate
- Physiotherapy to keep airways clear of mucus
- Encourage fluid intake to keep secretions moist
- Artificial ventilatory support.

Ask the patient about dietary habits as a high meat diet and starvation will cause a lowered urine pH.

If ketoacidosis is caused by newly diagnosed or unstable diabetes mellitus, insulin therapy will need to be started and adjusted until the body is in balance. The patient will then need to take over their own care before discharge, to secure the continuation of the new regime.

The acid urine may be due to infection of the urinary tract.

An uncontaminated urine specimen sent for culture and sensitivity will allow the bacteria to be isolated and an antibiotic found that would be effective against it.

In these circumstances the patient must be advised:
- To take the full course of antibiotics
- Take the antibiotics each day at the same time, without missing a dose
- To drink ample quantities of fluid.

URINE, PROTEIN

NORMAL MEASUREMENT

The urine should test negative for protein.

PROCEDURE

A urine reagent stick sensitive to protein, dipped into a clean specimen of urine.

Alkaline urine will cause the reagent stick to change colour.

Contaminants can alter results:
- Vaginal discharge
- Faeces
- Menstrual blood
- Poor hygiene.

PURPOSE

To detect the presence of protein in urine.

Red and white blood cells, plasma proteins and platelets, as the protein components of the blood, should not be detected in urine.

Proteins are normally not filtered into the renal tubule. Capillary blood vessels enter the glomerular cup of each of the two million nephrons (one million in each kidney). The filtering surface of the glomerulus has pores through which blood components enter the nephron. The size of the pores regulates the size of the molecules that are able to pass from the blood into the nephron.

The nephron is where urine is produced. If a substance is unable to enter the nephron, it can not be excreted in the urine.

Protein molecules are too large to enter the kidney nephrons through the glomerular pores. They remain in the capillary blood passing to the venous blood vessels that lead away from the kidneys.

Smaller proteins that can pass through the pores into the kidney nephron are quickly returned to the blood circulation through the nephron wall.

When these kidney mechanisms positively excluding protein from the urine become defective, proteins enter the nephrons. They pass through the nephron to be excreted in the urine.

As part of their normal function, nephrons will add a small amount of protein to the urine.

RAISED VALUES

PRESENCE OF PROTEIN IN THE URINE

Proteinuria

Renal disease
– Defective glomerular filtration
– Damage to tubules causing an excessive secretion of protein.

Renal distress
– Shock

Raised renal blood pressure
– Hypertension

Urinary tract disorders
– Urinary tract infection
– Haematuria

Raised temperature

Heart failure

Orthostatic or postural proteinuria
– A proteinuria presenting in children and adolescence, after they have been
  standing or exercising.
  It does not indicate disease.

Pre-eclampsia in pregnancy

ASSOCIATED INVESTIGATIONS

		Related pages
Temperature	A urinary tract infection will cause proteinuria. This may cause a rise in temperature.	4
Blood pressure	Hypertension may be associated with proteinuria.	17
Early morning urine test for protein, for comparison with test for protein later in the day	Orthostatic proteinuria will cause the morning urine to test negative to protein after lying horizontal in bed. Urine tested later after body position becomes upright will be positive for protein.	189
Routine testing of urine with reagent stick	To reveal the abnormal presence or abnormal concentrations of other substances in the urine.	174
A sterile urine specimen for culture and sensitivity	A urinary tract infection will cause proteinuria.	294

Microscopic examination of the urine for:

Microalbuminuria	This will detect the presence of albumin molecules that are in amounts too small for detection by urine dipstick reagents.	
Red blood cells	These should not appear in the urine. They can present as cylindrical casts. The appearance and condition of the cells can help in establishing where the cells entered the system.	
White blood cells	The presence of white blood cells will be evidence of inflammation or infection in the renal system. White cells can also present as casts.	

Creatinine clearance Blood urea	Tests of renal function.	119 121
Daily weight	Substantial loss of plasma proteins will cause tissue oedema. A rapid gain in weight will reflect this.	264
Total protein values Albumin and globulin values	To see the effect that the lost protein has on the normal blood protein values.	75 77

CONSIDERATIONS FOR CARE

The effects of proteinuria on patients will depend on the amount of protein lost and the length of time that the condition continues.

When large amounts of protein from the blood are routinely lost in the urine, changes to the circulatory system will become apparent.

Protein provides the osmotic pull that attracts water back into the blood vessels from the body tissues.
As the amount of circulating proteins diminishes, the osmotic pull of the blood is reduced. Oedema becomes evident, and may become severe.

As with all oedematous tissue, the skin around it becomes weakened, stretched and liable to injury. The waterlogged tissue and poor circulation prevents rapid healing. This skin must not have pressure applied to it. It must be kept clean and away from risk of injury.

Comfortable supportive positioning must take account of these factors.
Positioning in an upright position also becomes important when pulmonary oedema causes breathlessness.

Daily weighing will monitor the retention or reduction of oedematous fluid.

This loss of fluid from the circulating volume will mean a reduced renal blood flow. Urinary output will diminish. A fluid input and output chart will be needed to keep this situation under review.

An increasing pulse rate and a lowered blood pressure will also reflect a reduction in the volume of circulating blood.

Each urine specimen should be tested for protein and the degree of loss recorded.

Intravenous infusions of albumin may be given to replace the lost protein.

Diuretic therapy will reduce the oedema and increase blood flow to the kidneys. They may also bring further hypovolaemia, so the fluid status of the patient must be monitored continually.

The patient will feel lethargic and unwell. Hypovolaemia may cause postural hypotension.
Despite this, gentle exercise will be important to prevent thrombosis, a risk heightened by the low circulating volume.

Gamma globulins are also lost through the kidneys.
The loss of these immunoglobulins weakens the body's defences against infections. Prevention and early recognition of infectious states will become important.

A rise in temperature or the development of pain, cough or inflammation will be significant.

URINE, GLUCOSE

NORMAL MEASUREMENT

The urine should test negative for glucose.

PROCEDURE

Urine testing reagent stick for glucose.

The urine specimen should be fresh when tested.

To obtain an accurate glycosuria measurement, the specimen for testing should be taken one hour after the patient has previously emptied his or her bladder.

The first specimen of the morning will not give an accurate measurement of glucose present in the urine.

PURPOSE

To test for the presence of glucose in the urine.

Although glucose enters the kidney nephrons, it is normally completely reabsorbed back into the blood circulation. Glucose does not enter the urine.

The reabsorption of glucose by the nephron is limited by the ability of the cells along the walls of the tubule to transport glucose out of the nephron and back into the circulation.

When every means of glucose transport through the nephron wall is full to capacity, the 'renal threshold' has been reached. If, at that stage, a quantity of glucose remains in the nephron and is unable to be absorbed, it continues through the nephron to be excreted in the urine. The urine then tests positive for glucose.

This situation occurs when the amount of circulating glucose is high and excessive amounts of glucose are entering the kidney tubules.

The limit set by the renal threshold varies with each individual.

Glucose is an osmotic diuretic. Glucose attracts and pulls water along its path.

The presence of glucose in the urine will mean an increase in urine volume.

RAISED VALUES

PRESENCE OF GLUCOSE IN URINE

Glycosuria

False positive
– Hypochlorite cleaner in urine flask
– Large amounts of vitamin C

Raised blood glucose
– During the first 2 hours after a meal
– Diabetes mellitus
– Cushing's syndrome
– Adrenal disorders
– Raised intracranial pressure
– Phaeochromocytoma

Lowered renal threshold
– Pregnancy
– Eclampsia

Defective absorption mechanism in renal tubules
– Fanconi's syndrome

Effects of drugs, including:
– Corticosteroids
– Indometacin
– Thiazide diuretics

ASSOCIATED INVESTIGATIONS

		Related pages
Blood glucose	Glucose is excreted in the urine when the blood glucose is elevated.	**85**
Glucose tolerance test	A test to monitor blood glucose values, following a measured intake of glucose.	
Urine test for ketones	When cells are unable to use glucose as a metabolic fuel, the liver converts fats for use in its place. This process produces ketones as a by-product. They are excreted in the urine.	**197**
Urine pH	Ketones are acids. A raised ketone value in the blood and the urine will lower their pH.	**184** **150**
Respirations	A lowered blood pH value will increase the respiratory rate. Exhaled air may smell of acetone.	**129**
Fluid input and output chart	Glucose has an osmotic pull. When the quantity of glucose excreted through the kidney is high, the amount of water excreted with it will also be raised. Fluid intake will be increased to compensate the loss.	
Signs of dehydration	If the amount of water lost through the kidneys is not fully replaced, the body will become dehydrated.	
Level of consciousness	Glycosuria reflects a rise in blood sugar. The brain reacts badly when it has excessive amounts of glucose entering its cells. Hyperglycaemia will gradually bring about unconsciousness.	**262**
Signs of infection	Infection risks are higher when a state of hyperglycaemia exists.	

CONSIDERATIONS FOR CARE

Most patients know that when they give a specimen of urine for routine testing, it will be checked for 'sugar'. They also know that urine which tests positive for glucose can be a sign of diabetes mellitus. Care and tact are needed when informing a patient that glucose has been found in their urine, as the information can be distressing.

Conclusions can not be drawn from a single specimen that tests positive to glucose. Further investigations will be needed.

The presence of glucose need not signify diabetes mellitus; other causes are possible.

Glycosuria can be a temporary condition. It may appear after a meal or when the glucose renal threshold is reduced in pregnancy. Once the temporary nature of the glycosuria is confirmed no further action will be needed.

If diabetes mellitus is confirmed, the points of care for a raised blood glucose (page 90) will apply.

Glycosuria can be the result of raised circulating glucocorticoids, caused either by disease or drug therapy, Cushing's disease or Cushing's syndrome. Proteins will then be used as an energy source for cells in place of glucose – gluconeogenesis. Blood glucose values will rise until glucose appears in the urine. The glycosuria will resolve when there is a reduction in steroid therapy or resolution of the Cushing's disease.

NORMAL MEASUREMENT

The urine should test negative for ketones.

PROCEDURE

A fresh specimen of urine should be tested.

A ketone reagent urine test stick.

PURPOSE

To test for the presence of ketones in the urine.

Ketone bodies are formed when stored fats are used to produce energy in place of carbohydrates (glyconeogenesis).

The ketone bodies are:
- Acetone
- Beta hydroxybutyric acid
- Acetoacetic acid.

Ketones are products generated by the liver. They are the fuels derived from fats that can be used by the cells to produce energy.

Ketones are taken into cells, where they enter the energy-producing pathways in place of glucose.

Myocardial cells favour acetoacetic acid in preference to glucose for energy generation.

Brain cells are unable to use ketones as a fuel. They rely on glucose alone.

Carbohydrate metabolism is disrupted:
- By lack of carbohydrates in the diet
- When the body is unable to convert the dietary carbohydrates into glucose
- Fat stores are mobilised to take the place of glucose as an energy-generating fuel.

Hormonal factors stimulate the conversion of excessive amounts of fat. The unused ketones remain in the blood circulation (ketoacidosis). This can lead to a lowering of the body pH.

Ketone bodies appear in the urine when ketone production exceeds their use. Ketones are strong acids to expel through the urine so sodium is also expelled with them as a neutralising agent. The loss of sodium from the blood and tissue fluid means that this positive ion has to be replaced with another positive ion and positive hydrogen ions are utilised. The acidosis therefore becomes worse.

NORMAL PHYSIOLOGY

Carbohydrates usually provide the body with its food source for energy.

Dietary proteins and fats are taken in excess.

They are stored in fat stores as a supplementary source of energy.

When carbohydrate is not available for use and blood glucose values are low, fat stores are mobilised as an alternative source of energy for cell metabolism.

Hormone changes that result in gluconeogenesis cause the reaction to be in excess of body needs.

Excess proteins, carbohydrates and fats are stored in adipose tissues. They are stored in the form of triglycerides.

When needed, the triglycerides are broken down into fatty acids for transport in the blood to the liver.
The fatty acids re-form to triglycerides before they are used by the liver cells.

In the liver, the triglycerides split into: fatty acids and glycerol

The liver keeps some fatty acids for its own use.

Glycerol is easily absorbed into the glucose pathways to provide energy where it is needed.

Other fatty acids are converted to the ketone acetone for transport in blood to other tissues, providing a fuel source for energy production.

The ketones beta hydroxybutyric acid and acetoacetic acid are also formed in the liver.

As this response to failed glucose metabolism is surplus to actual need, the liver continues to manufacture ketones beyond the capacity of cells to use them all.

Blood ketone levels rise.

Ketones appear in the urine.

Small amounts of acetone are excreted through the lungs, with expiration.

RAISED VALUES

PRESENCE OF KETONES IN URINE

Lack of dietary intake of carbohydrates
– Malnutrition
– Dieting
– High fat or protein diet

Disorders of carbohydrate metabolism
– Decreased insulin production, diabetes mellitus
– Glycogen storage disease
– Ketoacidosis

Rapid use of fat stores
– Speedy weight loss
– Cold exposure
– Strenuous exercise
– Febrile illness
– Increased metabolic rate

Pregnancy

Eclampsia

Increased production from pituitary gland
– Corticotrophic hormone
– Growth hormone

Increased secretion of cortisone from adrenal cortex

Drugs giving a false-positive result
– Levodopa
– Pyridium

ASSOCIATED INVESTIGATIONS

		Related pages
Blood glucose level	Undiagnosed or unstable diabetes mellitus can	**85**
Test urine for glucose	cause the urine to test positive for ketones.	**193**
Blood pH	Ketones are very acid. When they occur in excess	**150**
Urine pH	in the blood, the body pH falls and produces a state of acidosis. The excretion of ketones in the urine lowers the urine pH and it becomes more acid.	**184**
Respirations	Metabolic acidosis will cause an increase in respiration rate and depth, in an attempt to decrease the hydrogen ion content of the blood.	**129**
Smell of acetone on the breath	A raised blood ketone concentration will cause the breath to smell of acetone.	
Electrolyte values in blood ■ Sodium ■ Potassium ■ Chloride ■ Bicarbonate	Ketoacidosis will cause movements of electrolytes, in an attempt to redress the electrical and acid–base balance of the body. Dehydration, polyuria and vomiting will cause further electrolyte imbalance.	**97** **102** **107**
Signs of dehydration	If the ketones in the urine are due to a raised blood glucose, excretion of excess glucose through the kidneys will force an osmotic diuresis. Vomiting may accompany ketoacidosis with further loss of fluids.	
Pulse	A raised pulse and lowered blood pressure will	**9**
Blood pressure	indicate hypovolaemia from a high fluid output.	**17**
Levels of consciousness	Acidosis if unchecked will cause coma and death. Hyperglycaemia, which may precipitate the manufacture of ketones, can also cause a diminishing level of consciousness.	**262**

CONSIDERATIONS FOR CARE

It is the acidic nature of ketones that makes them harmful. Body pH must be kept within very narrow limits. Buffering systems in the blood are effective in reducing the harmful effects of ketones, but once all the buffers have been used and the compensatory mechanisms have reached their limits, blood pH will alter and life is threatened.

The production of ketones, and their appearance in the urine, can often be easily explained. Temporary loss of appetite, fever, an acute episode of vomiting are all occasions when the body's intake of glucose is reduced or temporarily stopped, or glucose stores are depleted.

Glyconeogenesis of fats will provide energy during this short glucose gap.

Once the dietary intake of glucose is resumed, the ketones will disappear.

Alternative routes using intravenous or nasogastric tube administration will be needed if glucose can not be taken orally.

The condition may arise, as with diabetes mellitus, that the body becomes unable to metabolise glucose for its energy needs. Glyconeogenesis will then produce ketones in large amounts over a prolonged period. A state of ketoacidosis will develop.

Vomiting caused by the state of acidosis will further dehydrate the patient and cause increased electrolyte imbalance.

Therapy to activate glucose metabolism will be needed to stop the process of ketone production.

Correction of fluid and electrolyte imbalances will also be necessary.

Each urine specimen must be collected and tested to record the quantity of ketones excreted.

NORMAL MEASUREMENT

The urine should test negative for blood.

PROCEDURE

A fresh specimen of urine should be used.

A blood reagent urine dipstick.

False-positive results originate from:
- Traces of hypochlorite cleaning solution in the collecting container
- A menstruating woman.

PURPOSE

To test for the presence of red blood cells, free haemoglobin or free myoglobin in the urine.

The colour of the urine will change from normal yellow to red, as the amount of blood contained in the urine increases. Food dyes, beetroot or acute porphyria may also colour the urine red.

Urine tests for blood differentiate between 'haemolysed' and 'non-haemolysed' blood.

Non-haemolysed blood	The reagent stick is identifying intact red blood cells in the urine.
Haemolysed blood	The reagent stick is identifying free haemoglobin or myoglobin in the urine. These products escape from red blood cells when they break down or rupture.

Red blood cells should not be part of urine formation. If, through disease, they enter the urinary pathways, they will become damaged or misshapen by the environment. The osmotic pressure exerted by the contents of the red blood cell in a dilute urine will cause the cell to absorb water until the cell wall bursts. Haemoglobin will be released and the urine will test positively for haemolysed blood. Passage through the narrow nephrons will also damage red blood cells.

The condition of the red blood cells may therefore give some indication of the point at which red blood cells entered the urinary tract.

Non-haemolysed red blood cells	The good condition of these red cells suggests that they entered low down the urinary tract, i.e. from the prostate gland.
Haemolysed red blood cells	The poor survival of the red blood cell suggests that bleeding took place higher in the urinary tract, i.e. the renal tubules.

The presence of red blood cell casts in the urine will confirm bleeding into the renal tubules. These are microscopic cylinders of red blood cells that are formed when tubules are inflamed, infected or are degenerating. They are washed out in the urine.

RAISED VALUES

THE PRESENCE OF BLOOD IN THE URINE (HAEMATURIA)

Kidney disease
– Inflammatory
– Infectious
– Neoplastic disease
– Stones

Ureteric disease
– Stones
– Neoplasm

Bladder
– Neoplasm
– Stones
– Cystitis

Prostate gland
– Prostatitis
– Neoplasm

Urethra
– Urethritis

Trauma to any part of the urinary tract
– Following suprapubic aspiration

Anticoagulation therapy

Transfusion reactions

Menstruation

Following extrarenal red cell damage and haemolysis, haemoglobin can be
excreted through the urine
– Trauma
– Post-operative

Myoglobin released after muscle damage and excreted in the urine
– Strenuous exercise

ASSOCIATED INVESTIGATIONS

		Related pages
Microscopic examination of the urine	To positively identify the presence of red blood cells in the urine. To examine the condition of the red blood cells. To look for casts of red blood cells as evidence of renal tubule disease. Microscopy will also show the presence of white blood cells, albumin and bacteria.	
Test urine for protein	Protein presents in the urine when there is disease of the renal tubule. When protein appears in the urine in addition to haematuria, it can indicate that the kidneys are the source of the haematuria.	189
A sterile specimen of urine for culture and sensitivity	A urinary tract infection may cause haematuria.	294
Throat swab for culture and sensitivity	A glomerular nephritis can occur after a streptococcal throat infection.	
Blood haemoglobin Red blood cell count	To ensure that the blood loss through the urinary tract has not caused anaemia.	38 34
White blood cell count	A raised white cell count would indicate that an inflammatory or infectious process was active in the urinary tract.	44
Blood pressure	Reduced renal function will increase blood pressure. A raised blood pressure in the presence of haematuria will provide evidence of renal disease.	17
Serum creatinine Blood urea	These tests are used to monitor kidney function.	119 121
Renal and urinary tract imaging tests	■ Ultrasound examination ■ X-ray ■ Renal arteriography ■ Intravenous pyelography ■ Computerised tomography ■ Micturating cystourography ■ Renal scintigraphy	298 295 296

CONSIDERATIONS FOR CARE

The appearance of visible blood in the urine is a disconcerting experience. Until a benign reason for its presence is found, it will remain a source of anxiety.

If the loss of blood causes anaemia, this must be corrected. The feeling of tiredness and lethargy that comes from anaemia will compound the feelings of ill-health that are produced by renal disease.

When haematuria has its source in the glomeruli, or disease of the renal tubules, it is essential that renal function is assessed constantly. The fluid balance of the body must be kept under constant surveillance, to monitor the degree of renal dysfunction:

- Accurate fluid intake and output recordings
- Daily weighings, at the same time of day, wearing the same clothes
- Observe for signs of oedematous tissues.

If the urine output is poor and fluid retention is evident, the daily fluid intake will be restricted to: the previous day's output + 500 ml to compensate for invisible fluid loss.

Regular frequent blood pressure measurement will also be required. This is liable to become elevated as:

- The restricted excretion of fluids through the kidney will increase the circulating volume
- Sodium excretion will be reduced. The increased sodium increases the osmotic pull, attracting excess water to the tissues and increasing the circulating volume.

Complete rest is recommended.

Attention to skin and pressure areas will be needed if oedema is present.

All urine should be tested for blood and protein, and the results recorded in a chronological pattern. This will give some indication of the diseased state of the glomeruli and tubules.

The source of haematuria may be found lower down the urinary tract. When infection is suspected, it is useful to obtain a urine specimen for culture to isolate the causative bacteria before antibiotic therapy begins.

The care given should be centred on alleviating the discomforts of this condition until the inflammation resolves:

- Warm baths will ease perineal discomfort
- Copious drinks dilute the urine and wash the infectious material and debris through the urinary tract. This also gives some protection against infection tracking upwards towards the kidneys.

URINE, NITRITE AND LEUCOCYTES

NORMAL MEASUREMENT

The urine should test negative for nitrites and leucocytes.

PROCEDURE

A reagent stick sensitive to nitrites and leucocytes dipped into a fresh specimen of urine.

The urine must have been in the bladder for at least 3 hours.

PURPOSE

To measure the nitrite and leucocyte values in a specimen of urine.

A urinary tract infection causes a rise in measured nitrite and leucocytes in the urine.

Urine normally contains nitrates as a waste product of protein breakdown. Some strains of bacteria have an enzyme that will break down the nitrate to nitrite as the urine collects in the bladder. The expelled urine will have a raised nitrite level when tested.

Some bacteria have no metabolic action on nitrates. The test will not recognise the presence of a urinary tract infection in these circumstances.

The presence of a urinary tract infection causes an inflammatory response. This will increase the presence of white blood cells. The leucocyte count, and the presence of damaged leucocytes, in the urine will rise and these white blood cells will release leucocyte esterase which can be measured by testing.

Casts in urine

Microscopic examination of the urine may show casts. They are aggregates of protein formed in the nephron or collecting duct of the renal tubule when renal disease is present. There are various forms of cast associated with renal disease but acidic conditions with decreased urine flow, and the presence of protein and sodium, are needed for their formation.

Crystal formations in urine

Renal damage or disease should be suspected if excessive crystal formation causes the urine to become cloudy. Crystal formations appearing in the urine as an end product of food metabolism will not indicate disease.

Bilirubin changes structure as it passes along physiological pathways.

Methods of measurement will change, depending on the form of bilirubin that needs estimation:
- Serum bilirubin – measure the circulating levels of unconjugated bilirubin and conjugated bilirubin
- Urine urobilinogen – urine should test negative to urobilinogen
- Urine bilirubin – bilirubin is not normally found in the urine.

Abnormal test results occur when disease alters the normal sequence of changes by bilirubin.

The combination of abnormal values will often mark where disruption of the normal pathway is occurring.

Knowledge of the events and changes affecting bilirubin help to clarify the effects of disease on the biliary system.

Bilirubin is a golden-coloured pigment. This colour is most obviously seen when the skin is recovering from a bruise. The collected red blood cells haemolyse and bilirubin is a product of this breakdown. The bruise will turn from red/blue to yellow. A rise in circulating serum bilirubin may cause a general yellowing of skin colour and sclera of the eyes – jaundice.

A rise in urine bilirubin will darken the urine colour.

DIRECT AND INDIRECT BILIRUBIN

Conjugated bilirubin may be referred to as direct bilirubin and unconjugated bilirubin as indirect bilirubin. The terms originate from the van den Bergh's test of serum bilirubin.

Conjugated bilirubin gives a direct reaction to the test reagents. Unconjugated bilirubin needs modification prior to testing and is said to be indirectly tested.

NORMAL PHYSIOLOGY

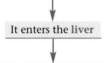

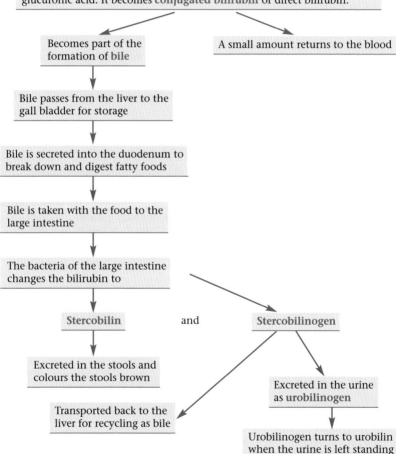

Red blood cells destroyed by the reticulo-endothelial system release bilirubin into the blood.
Bilirubin travels attached to plasma proteins as unconjugated bilirubin or indirect bilirubin.

It enters the liver

The enzyme glucuronyl transferase causes the bilirubin to conjugate with glucuronic acid. It becomes conjugated bilirubin or direct bilirubin.

Becomes part of the formation of bile

A small amount returns to the blood

Bile passes from the liver to the gall bladder for storage

Bile is secreted into the duodenum to break down and digest fatty foods

Bile is taken with the food to the large intestine

The bacteria of the large intestine changes the bilirubin to

Stercobilin   and   Stercobilinogen

Excreted in the stools and colours the stools brown

Transported back to the liver for recycling as bile

Excreted in the urine as urobilinogen

Urobilinogen turns to urobilin when the urine is left standing

ASSOCIATED INVESTIGATIONS

		Related pages
Red blood cell count and haemoglobin	Bilirubin is derived from haemoglobin when red blood cells are destroyed.	34 38
White blood cell count	A change in the values of the differential white blood count may identify the cause, when the ability of the liver to process bile is disrupted.	44
Plasma albumin	Albumin is manufactured by the liver. When liver function is seriously diminished, albumin values fall.	75
Plasma globulin	Chronic liver disease stimulates the immune system, causing a rise in the blood globulin concentration.	77
Prothrombin time	Formed in the liver, a lengthening prothrombin time will be significant when assessing the liver's ability to function.	66
Faecal fat measurement	The absence of bile will prevent the digestion and absorption of fat in the small intestine. The consequence of this will be steatorrhoea.	167
Aspartate aminotransferase (AST)	Also known as SGOT. The value rises in direct relation to the amount of liver tissue that is damaged.	
Alanine transferase	An enzyme that is produced when liver cells become damaged.	
Visual imaging of the liver and biliary tracts	▪ Ultrasound scan ▪ Computerised tomography ▪ Cholangiography ▪ Endoscopic retrograde cholangiopancreatography	298 296
Liver biopsy	Microscopic examination of the liver cells.	

CONSIDERATIONS FOR CARE

A steep elevation in unconjugated serum bilirubin carries the risk of kernicterus.

As a consequence of foetal life, the newborn baby has an excessive number of red blood cells. The surplus cells are destroyed in the days following delivery. The effect of this can be to produce a physiological jaundice, the yellowing of the skin caused by a rise in unconjugated bilirubin. If the unconjugated bilirubin blood value exceeds acceptable limits, the baby becomes at risk of kernicterus. Ensuring that the mother is supported to give sufficient feeds to the baby prevents dehydration during this time. Excessively high values of serum bilirubin are treated with phototherapy or exchange transfusions.

The excessive destruction of red blood cells due to disease will cause anaemia. The oxygen-carrying component of the blood will be diminished. The patient will experience lethargy, breathlessness and tachycardia.

A raised conjugated serum bilirubin may be a sign that bile is not entering the duodenum. Fat will not be digested or absorbed.

As a consequence of this the patient can feel:
- Flatulent
- A discomfort and intolerance of fatty food
- Loss of appetite
- Nauseous.

A reduced fat diet will be required.

The loss of absorbed fat will reduce the amount of vitamin K available for the production of prothrombin. Blood will take longer to clot.

Vitamin K supplements will be needed prior to surgery.

Jaundice can be an uncomfortable condition. Pruritis may be a problem.

Light clothes, a cool room and comforting baths may help the patient feel easier.

The patient will need support to help them come to terms with the change in their appearance.

They may be embarrassed and worried about the cause of this change.

Explanations in terms that the patient can understand will be essential.

REFERENCE RANGE

Conjugated bilirubin (direct) – Adult: <17 µmol/l

                                 Child: 1.7–20.5mmol/l

                                 Neonate: 4–17 µmol/l

PROCEDURE

Venepuncture.

Raised concentrations of serum bilirubin may make the blood clotting mechanism less effective. The puncture site will then need prolonged compression to stop bleeding.

Immediate dispatch to the laboratory, as light will cause the bilirubin to break down.

Damage or haemolysis of the red blood cells will artificially raise the serum bilirubin.

The specimen must be handled carefully.

CONTAINER

The specimen container used in this unit is:

PURPOSE

To measure the concentration of unconjugated and conjugated bilirubin in the blood.

Unconjugated bilirubin (indirect)

Unconjugated bilirubin is bilirubin circulating in the blood attached to plasma proteins. When all plasma protein transport sites are full it will travel as free bilirubin. It has been produced by the breakdown of red blood cells. It has not been processed in the liver to form the bilirubin found in bile.

Unconjugated bilirubin has the ability to pass through the membranes of the brain cells. High levels of unconjugated bilirubin will cause permanent damage to the neurons, a condition termed kernicterus.

For neonates, the physiological breakdown of red blood cells following birth, together with the immaturity of the liver, can cause a rise in the serum levels of unconjugated bilirubin.

Conjugated bilirubin (direct)

Bilirubin is conjugated in the liver enabling it to become active in bile. A little conjugated bilirubin is usually in the blood. Liver and bile duct disease may cause the backtrack of conjugated bilirubin into the blood and a rise of the serum value. This usually reduces the amount of bile available to act on the fat in the intestine.

The consequences of this will be:
- The stools will have a high fat content
- The stools will be pale due to lack of bile pigment
- Blood clotting times will be lengthened. Vitamin K as a fat-soluble vitamin is necessary for prothrombin formation. The decrease in absorbed fat will reduce the available vitamin K and subsequently prothrombin values.

Bilirubin will be excreted in the urine causing the urine to become dark.

The skin and the sclera of the eyes will become jaundiced. Conjugated bilirubin does not pass through the membranes of brain cells. It will not cause kernicterus.

RAISED VALUES

HYPERBILIRUBINAEMIA

Raised values of *unconjugated* bilirubin

Excessive breakdown of red blood cells:
– Haemolytic disease
– Incompatible blood transfusion causing red cell haemolysis
– Resolution of internal haemorrhage
– Physiological haemolysis in the newborn.

Deficiency in the action of enzyme glucuronyl transferase to convert unconjugated bilirubin to conjugated bilirubin:
– Glucuronyl transferase disease of the newborn.

Liver disease interrupting the formation of bile:
– Infection
– Inflammation.

Raised values of *conjugated* bilirubin

Liver disease causing swelling of hepatic tissue. This blocks the pathways of bile into the biliary tracts:
– Infections
– Inflammation
– Auto-immune disease
– Cirrhosis.

Obstruction of the biliary pathways:
– Tumours
– Stones
– Inflammation of the gall bladder
– Outside pressure blocking the biliary tubes.

NORMAL MEASUREMENT

The urine should test negative for urobilinogen.

PROCEDURE

Urine urobilinogen reagent stick.

The urine must be fresh when tested.

Light will degrade the urobilinogen.

24-hour specimen containers must be kept in a dark place when making a urine collection.

If hepatitis is suspected, preventive measures must be taken to avoid the spread of infection:
- Protective clothing
- Warning label on specimens.

PURPOSE

To measure the amount of urobilinogen in the urine.

Urobilinogen degrades to urobilin when the urine is left to stand.

Levels of urine urobilinogen are at their highest during the afternoon and evening.

Conjugated bile leaves the large intestine either:
- In the stools
- Or it enters the blood through the intestinal mucosa.

The bile pigments that have left the intestine are carried in the blood as urobilinogen.

Urobilinogen either:
- Returns to the liver to be recycled through the biliary pathways
- Is filtered through the kidney to be excreted in the urine.

Bilirubin does not usually appear in the urine.

A rise in conjugated serum bilirubin will cause bilirubin to appear in the urine.

Unconjugated bilirubin is unable to pass through the kidney and produce a positive test for bilirubin.

A jaundiced patient with a negative urine test for bilirubin indicates that the yellow skin colouring is caused by an excess of unconjugated bilirubin.

ALTERED VALUES

RAISED VALUES	LOWERED VALUES
Increased production of bilirubin From excessive breakdown of red blood cells – Haemolytic anaemia – Incompatible blood transfusion – Genetic disease	Anaemia A reduction in the quantity of haemoglobin released from which bilirubin is formed
	Obstruction of the biliary pathways – Tumours – Stones – Inflammation of the gall bladder – Outside pressure blocking the tubes
Increased action of bacteria in the large intestine – Increase in the quantity of bowel flora – Slow transit time through the intestine	Decreased action of bacteria in the large intestine – Antibiotics reducing the quantity of bowel flora – Diarrhoea, decreasing the transit time through the intestine
Decreased reabsorption of urobilinogen by the liver – Liver damage – Early hepatitis	Liver disease preventing the formation of conjugated bilirubin or bile – Absence of glucuronyl transferase – Infectious hepatitis – Inflammatory disease – Auto-immune disease
Alkaline urine increases the measured levels of urobilinogen	Acid urine decreases the measured levels of urobilinogen
False-positive results obtained from – Eating bananas – Effects of drugs, including: – Chlorpromazine	False-negative results obtained when the specimen of urine is not fresh when tested

REFERENCE RANGE

0–4 ng/ml

PROCEDURE

Venepuncture.

Provide an interval of 2 weeks between internal, urethral examination and the test.

CONTAINER

The specimen container used in this unit is:

PURPOSE

To determine whether there is a rise in the blood value of prostate specific antigen.

Prostate specific antigen (PSA) is manufactured by the epithelial cells of the prostate gland.

Although a raised PSA value is used as a tumour marker for prostatic adeno-carcinoma, PSA values may also be raised when the prostate is healthy or if benign hyperplasia of the prostate is present. Its non-specificity means that it can only be used as part of a range of diagnostic interventions when assessing the health of a prostate.

ASSOCIATED INVESTIGATIONS

*Related
pages*

Urine volume and flow	An enlarged prostate gland will interrupt the flow of urine through the urethra.	
Rectal examination	Palpation of the prostate gland.	
Transrectal ultrasonography	Imaging of the prostate.	

Sequential testing of these cardiac enzymes will monitor the extent, and progress, of a myocardial infarction.

Labelling each blood sample with time and date is essential.

CREATINE PHOSPHOKINASE (CPK)

REFERENCE RANGE

Adult: 38–170 iu/l

Child: 50–185 iu/l

Neonate: 44–1150 iu/l

PROCEDURE

Venepuncture.

CONTAINER

The specimen container used in this unit is:

PURPOSE

To assess the creatine phosphokinase content of the blood.

Creatine phosphokinase is an enzyme found in the heart, skeletal muscle and brain. When damage occurs to these tissues, creatine phosphokinase is leaked into the blood initiating an elevated value. Creatine phosphokinase can be further divided into isoenzymes, MB, MM and BB. These isoenzymes provide markers to identify the source of damaged tissue. A rise in MB-CPK will signify myocardial damage. Regular monitoring of CPK values will give an indication of the disease process.

ASPARATE AMINOTRANSFERASE (AST)

REFERENCE RANGE

Adult: 5–30 iu/l

Child: 25–75 iu/l

Neonate: 20–75 iu/l

PROCEDURE

Venepuncture.

CONTAINER

The specimen container used in this unit is:

PURPOSE

To assess the aspartate aminotransferase content of the blood.

The enzyme aspartate aminotransferase is found in the mitochondria of many tissues, including the liver and heart.

When cell injury occurs, causing inflammation or necrosis, aspartate amino-transferase is released into the tissues and blood values of the enzyme will rise. The rise in value will reflect the extent of the tissue damage.

Aspartate aminotransferase has a half life of 17 hours so the blood test is time critical.

LACTIC DEHYDROGENASE (LDH)

REFERENCE RANGE

Adult: 240–525 iu/l

Neonate: 357–953 iu/l

PROCEDURE

Venepuncture.

CONTAINER

The specimen container used in this unit is:

PURPOSE

To assess the lactate dehydrogenase content of the blood.

Lactate dehydrogenase is a component of most body organs, so a rise in LDH blood value is not specific to damage to heart muscle. It is the rise in its isoenzyme LDH_1 that provides the specific marker of myocardial damage.

ASSOCIATED INVESTIGATIONS

		Related pages
Pulse	An assessment of the rate, rhythm and volume of the heart beat.	9
Blood pressure	Damage to the myocardium will affect cardiac output.	17
Blood cholesterol values		127
Auscultation of the heart	Examination of the heart using a stethoscope to detect abnormalities of the pumping mechanism.	
Electrocardiogram	Denotes changes in the conduction of electrical impulses through the myocardium.	
Exercise electrocardiography Imaging techniques	Shows the response of the heart to exercise.	
Echocardiography	Using ultrasound technique, a picture of the moving heart will show size, structure and motion.	
Nuclear magnetic resonance imaging		
Chest X-ray	Shows the size and shape of the heart.	
Cardiac angiography	An X-ray sensitive medium is injected into the blood vessels of the heart to enable the blood flow through the cardiac vessels to be visualised. Abnormalities may include abnormal direction of blood flow, occlusion to flow, abnormalities of the blood vessels and abnormal tissue growth.	
Cardiac catheterisation	To give a picture of the cardiac chambers and blood vessels and provide pressure readings within the heart.	

LIVER FUNCTION TESTS

The value of aspartate aminotransferase (AST) is considered against the value of alanine aminotransferase (ALT) to differentiate between the causes of liver disease.

SERUM TRANSAMINASES

ASPARTATE AMINOTRANSFERASE (AST)

REFERENCE RANGE

Adult: 5–30 iu/l

Child: 25–75 iu/l

Neonate: 20–75 iu/l

PROCEDURE

Venepuncture.

CONTAINER

The specimen container used in this unit is:

PURPOSE

To assess the aspartate aminotransferase content of the blood.

The enzyme aspartate aminotransferase is found in the mitochondria of many tissues, including the liver and heart.

When cell injury occurs, causing inflammation or necrosis, aspartate aminotransferase is released into the tissues and blood values of the enzyme will rise.

The rise in value will reflect the extent of the tissue damage.

Aspartate aminotransferase has a half life of 17 hours so the blood test is time critical.

Sequential testing, in association with other liver enzyme markers, will chart the progress of the liver condition.

Alcoholic liver disease will raise the value of AST.

ALANINE AMINOTRANSFERASE (ALT)

REFERENCE RANGE

Adult: 5–30 iu/l

Child: 5–28 iu/l

Neonate: 9–44 iu/l

PROCEDURE

Venepuncture.

CONTAINER

The specimen container used in this unit is:

PURPOSE

To assess the alanine aminotransferase content of the blood.

A rise in the blood enzyme value of alanine aminotransferase is significant in both liver and myocardial disease.

It is found in the cytoplasm of liver and myocardial cells. If disease causes damage to these cells, alanine aminotransferase enters the tissues and blood.

ALT values rise with the inflammatory effects of hepatitis and obstructive biliary disease but the rise is less when a tumour is present.

ASSOCIATED INVESTIGATIONS

		Related pages
Serum bilirubin	The liver conjugates bilirubin, a breakdown product of red blood cells.	**211**
Urine bilirubin	This becomes a component of bile; manufactured by the liver, bile is secreted into the small intestine, for digestion of fat.	**207**
Urine urbilinogen	The blood values of conjugated and unconjugated bilirubin will indicate the ability of the liver to maintain this cycle of events.	**213**
Plasma proteins ■ Serum globulin ■ Serum albumin	The liver is the site of plasma protein manufacture. When the liver is failing in function, the plasma protein values will fall.	
Blood clotting time	The liver is the site of manufacture for components required for blood clotting. Blood clotting time will be extended if the liver fails in its function.	
Carbohydrate-deficient transferrin test	A test that identifies alcohol abuse and its effect on the liver.	
Serum amylase	Diagnostic of acute pancreatitis. As pancreatic cells become damaged or destroyed, amylase is released into the blood.	
Imaging of the liver	■ Ultrasound scan to detect masses and cysts. ■ Computerised tomography ■ Radioisotope liver scan.	
Tissue biopsy		

NORMAL PHYSIOLOGY

Ovum ripens in the ovary

↓

It comes to the surface of the ovary and is expelled from its Graffian follicle to be picked up by the fimbrae of the Fallopian tube

↓

Luteinizing hormone from the anterior pituitary gland causes the follicle to become the corpus luteum, a progesterone-secreting gland

↓

If unfertilised, the egg is expelled and the corpus luteum stops producing progesterone

If fertilised, the ovum will be taken into the uterus.
It will embed itself into the prepared endometrium.
The trophoblastic cells of the growing placenta start to secrete human chorionic gonadotrophin (hCG)

↓

hCG supports the continuing function of the corpus luteum

↓

Progesterone continues to be secreted and the pregnancy progresses

↓

Levels of hCG will fall when the placenta takes over full hormone production from the corpus luteum

Oestriols are placenta-generated oestrogens stimulated by substances produced by the liver and the adrenals of the foetus

↓

They are conjugated in the mother's liver

↓

They are excreted in the mother's urine

Alpha-foetal proteins are globulin proteins produced by the dividing cells of the foetal tissues

↓

The alpha-foetal proteins pass into the foetal circulation

↓

The alpha-foetal protein produced passes across the placental barrier into the mother's circulation

ASSOCIATED INVESTIGATIONS

		Related pages
Blood pressure	A rise in blood pressure is a sign of pre-eclampsia. Oedema and proteinuria are also associated with pre-eclampsia.	17
Examination for signs of oedema	Swollen face, fingers, ankles and feet.	283
Test urine for: ▪ Protein ▪ Glucose	Proteinuria (see above). Pregnancy lowers the renal threshold for glucose.	189 193
Weight	The gain in weight should be steady. The desired increase over the whole pregnancy should be about 10–12.6 kg. Excessive weight gain can be due to overeating or fluid retention. Insufficient weight gain may indicate a low birthweight baby.	264
Palpation of the abdomen	To measure the height of the enlarging abdomen. To feel the 'lie' of the baby in the uterus.	
Foetal heart rate	The heart rate of the foetus may be counted using a foetal stethoscope held to the abdomen or by using an electronic amplifying or sensing device.	
Haemoglobin Red blood cell count	The maternal blood volume increases with pregnancy. The number of blood cells and the amount of haemoglobin must also increase for blood values to remain normal.	38 34
Amniocentesis	A sample of amniotic fluid can be taken to test for foetal growth, maturity, disease, damage or distress.	
Pelvic ultrasound	An imaging technique for measuring foetal growth, confirming multiple pregnancies, investigating foetal abnormality.	298

HUMAN CHORIONIC GONADOTROPHIN (hCG)

REFERENCE RANGE

Non-pregnant serum value: <25 mU/l

Pregnancy: hCG values will vary according to gestation.

PROCEDURE

Venepuncture.

Urine specimen.

The serum test for hCG is more sensitive than the urine test.

A haemolysed specimen of blood will give a false result.

The test is ineffective after 20 weeks' gestation.

The test should be performed on an early morning specimen of urine.

CONTAINER

The specimen container used in this unit is:

PURPOSE

Measurements to assess hCG levels are usually taken to confirm pregnancy.

hCG is secreted by the placenta, following the fertilisation of an ovum.

It stimulates the production of progesterone from the corpus luteum until the placenta is able to take over hormone production for itself to maintain the pregnancy.

hCG is first produced 8–10 days after conception. Values continue to rise until they reach a peak at 8–12 weeks' gestation.

hCG values will not be significant after the 20th week of pregnancy.

As a test of pregnancy, the result of an hCG assessment will be very important.

The care and counselling that should follow this test will depend on the patient's satisfaction with the result.

ALTERED VALUES

RAISED VALUES	LOWERED VALUES
Pregnancy	Abortion
Some ectopic pregnancies	Ectopic pregnancy
Neoplasms – Hydatidiform moles – Chorionic carcinoma – Embryonal carcinoma – Pancreatic carcinoma – Malignant melanoma – Bronchogenic carcinoma – Breast – Testis	
Conditions that raise the ESR	
False positives – Haematuria or proteinuria – Soap contaminating the urine specimen	False negatives – Early pregnancy – Ectopic pregnancy – Very dilute urine
Effect of drugs, including: – Oral contraceptives	

SERUM ALPHA-FETOPROTEIN

REFERENCE RANGE

Non-pregnant state: 0–10 µg/l

PROCEDURE

Venepuncture.

Haemolysis of the red blood cells will alter the measured value. The specimen must be handled carefully.

CONTAINER

The specimen container used in this unit is:

PURPOSE

To measure the maternal alpha-fetoprotein value.

Alpha-fetoprotein is a globulin.

It is produced by the foetus as tissues develop from the midline region of the embryo, i.e. the liver and gastrointestinal tract. The protein passes across the placental barrier, from the foetal circulation to the maternal blood.

The value of alpha-fetoprotein will rise with foetal growth as the pregnancy progresses, then begins to fall in the final weeks.

Neural tube defects will cause a rise in the alpha-fetoprotein and the test is used to screen for these abnormalities.

The serum test results will then be used in combination with diagnostic values taken from an amniocentesis and ultrasound examination.

Alpha-fetoprotein is found in larger amounts in the amniotic fluid and will be part of the diagnostic values measured following amniocentesis.

Tumours causing cell division within the liver and other conditions can cause a rise in alpha-fetoprotein values in people who are not pregnant.

ALTERED VALUES

RAISED VALUES	LOWERED VALUES
Conditions related to pregnancy	
A fault in the physical development of the foetus	
– Neural tube defects, i.e. anencephaly, spina bifida, hydrocephalus	
– Oesophageal or duodenal atresia	
– Congenital abnormalities:	Down's syndrome
– Turner's syndrome	
– Congenital nephrosis	
– Cystic fibrosis	
– Fallot's tetralogy	
Threatened abortion	
Foetal distress	
Foetal death	
Multiple pregnancy	
Inaccurate estimated date of delivery	Inaccurate estimated date of delivery
Conditions unrelated to pregnancy	
Tumours of the liver	
– Hepatoma	
Tumours of the reproductive system	
– Tumour of the testes	
– Tumour of the ovaries	
Tumours of the gastrointestinal tract	
– Stomach	
– Biliary system	
– Pancreas	
Viral hepatitis	
Cirrhosis of the liver	
Ataxia-telangiectasia	

OESTRIOLS

REFERENCE RANGE

Varies with duration of pregnancy.

Please refer to local values.

PROCEDURE

Venepuncture.

24-hour urine collection.

CONTAINER

The specimen container used in this unit is:

PURPOSE

To measure the placental manufacture of oestriol.

Oestriol is produced by the placenta. It is manufactured in combination with substances produced by the foetal liver and adrenal cortex.

The secretion of oestriol increases as the foetus grows, raising the measured oestriol values as the pregnancy progresses.

Serial recording of oestriol values will give a good picture of placental function and the growth of the infant.

A fall in the oestriol values is a warning sign that there is a drop in placental efficiency.

This will be detrimental to the health and growth of the foetus. Consecutive falls in oestriol values will be an important factor when deciding when a pregnancy needs to be artificially curtailed.

ALTERED VALUES

RAISED VALUES	LOWERED VALUES
Multiple pregnancy	Placental insufficiency Abortion
Adreno-cortical hyperplasia Adreno-cortical tumour	Maternal liver dysfunction
Ovarian tumour	Maternal renal dysfunction during pregnancy – Diabetes mellitus – Hypertension
Testicular tumour	Maternal malnutrition
	Foetal abnormalities – Down's syndrome – Anencephaly

ASSOCIATED INVESTIGATIONS

LECITHIN/SPHINGOMYELIN RATIO

Lecithin is a component of surfactant, molecules produced in the alveolar membrane of the lung.

Sphingomyelin is produced by the membranes of the foetal lung.

As the ratio of lecithin production to sphingomyelin production is charted against gestational age, the maturity of the foetal lung and its ability to function following birth can be assessed.

AMNIOCENTESIS

A sample of the amniotic fluid that surrounds the baby is aspirated through a needle that has been passed through the abdominal wall of the pregnant woman. The amniotic fluid is examined for:
- Abnormal components, blood, meconium, bilirubin
- Chromosome analysis
- Indicators of congenital disease of the foetus, e.g. alpha-fetoprotein, acetylcholinesterase, are associated with neural tube defects
- Signs of rhesus incompatibility: the presence of unconjugated bilirubin from red blood cell destruction.

GUTHRIE TEST – SERUM PHENYLALANINE

REFERENCE RANGE

Below 25 mg/dl

PROCEDURE

Heel stab, to provide drops of blood that fall within designated circles on prescribed printed card.

If not stored appropriately, the test should be sent to the laboratory for testing without a prolonged delay.

Refer to local policies regarding the number of days that should elapse following birth and the timing of the test.

PURPOSE

To ensure that the blood phenylalanine value is not raised.

A raised phenylalanine value will also be detectable in the urine.

Phenylketonuria is an inborn error of metabolism for which all newborns should be screened before 7 days of life, provided that they have had oral milk feeds since birth.

The conversion of the amino acid phenylalanine to its next breakdown product, tyrosine, depends on the presence of the enzyme, phenylalanine hydroxylase. If this enzyme is absent, the conversion does not occur and unchanged phenyl-alanine begins to accumulate in the cells, tissues and blood. If undetected, damage will occur to the central nervous system leading to poor cognitive ability and epilepsy.

If the test proves positive for phenylketonuria, a low phenylalanine diet must be given to maintain the blood phenylalanine value between 4–8 mg/dl.

ALTERED VALUES

RAISED VALUES	LOWERED VALUES
Phenylketonuria	Test taken too early
Liver disease	Insufficient oral milk feeds
Immature liver	

REFERENCE RANGE

Each cell carries 23 pairs of chromosomes, the karyotype 22 pairs of autosomes and 1 pair of sex chromosomes.

PROCEDURE

Cells taken from blood, bone marrow or tissue.

CONTAINER

The specimen container used in this unit is:

PURPOSE

Genes are carried in the chromosome, providing the instructions for cell development and function.

They determine the structure and function of protein and it is the interaction of the proteins that make up our physical characteristics.

The foundation substance of genes is deoxyribonucleic acid (DNA). A chromosome is one coiled DNA molecule, supported by some structural protein. When the chromosome is uncoiled it looks like a ladder and it is the rungs of the ladder that are the 'bases' or nucleotides, which are the basic instructors or codes. Each chromosome has millions of bases.

Human chromosomes have a long 'q' arm and a short 'p' arm. They have a constriction called a centromere.

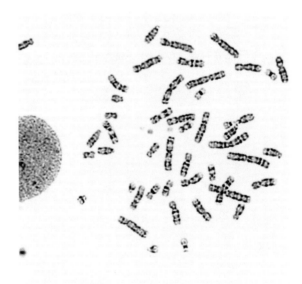

Source: P. Kumar and M. Clark, Clinical Medicine, 5th Edn, W.B. Saunders

Identification of a part of a chromosome uses the chromosome number and the arm descriptor, so designation 7q refers to the long arm of chromosome 7.

The expression of genes that make up a person is called a genotype. The observable characteristics of that person from the expression of those genes is called the phenotype.

Two genes that affect the same inherited trait, occupying corresponding sites on paired chromosomes, are called alleles. They may code for the same characteristic, or for different characteristics, following a pattern of expression described as dominant or recessive. The expression of the genes will also depend on other genes and the influence of the environment. Several genetic expressions may be involved with the development of a particular trait, e.g. height.

There are 3 categories of genetic conditions:
- Single gene
  - autosomal recessive disorder; both parents carry a single gene mutation for the disease to appear, i.e. sickle cell anaemia
  - single gene recessive disorder; one copy of the gene is transmitted by a parent
  - single gene X-linked: if the mutant gene is located on the X chromosome it will always be expressed in boys as the presence of a Y chromosome means that there is nothing to oppose it. Females with an X chromosome will have a normal gene to oppose it.
- Chromosomal disorders – This genetic disorder occurs during gamete development prior to conception. The number of chromosomes may not be normal (Down's syndrome) or the structure of the chromosome may be broken or translocated.
- Multifactorial inheritance – The effect of genetic patterning and the environment brings a predisposition to coronary heart disease or diabetes.

ANALYSIS

Cells are studied at the metaphase stage of mitosis when their patterning is most easily observed for analysis.

The chromosomes are stained and the organisation of their banding is studied for genetic re-arrangement or insertion, genetic mutations and deletions.

Gene and DNA sequencing can be analysed using more advanced technology. These tests can give a percentage risk of a condition appearing.

ASSOCIATED INVESTIGATIONS

Alpha-fetoprotein	Some congenital defects will raise alpha-fetoprotein values during pregnancy.
Ultrasound screening	Imaging of the growing foetus.
Chorionic villus biopsy	Collection of cells for analysis.
Amniocentesis	

CONSIDERATIONS FOR CARE

A thorough family history will be required to be used in association with the tests.

Before chromosome and genetic analysis takes place, discussion regarding the results must take place with the patient.

The test may reveal difficult information in terms of inheritance of disease and congenital conditions.

The calculation of percentage risk is a difficult concept and will need explanation.

Strict confidentiality must be kept at all times.

These tests should only be used to give further information on conditions that are under present consideration. They should only be used to predict future disease in rare circumstances.

CEREBROSPINAL FLUID

REFERENCE RANGE

Colourless fluid.

Volume – Adult: 150 ml fluid

Pressure – Adult: 40–180 mmH$_2$O

          – Child: 50–150 mmH$_2$O

PROCEDURE

Lumbar puncture:
- Supportive care must assist the patient to remain completely still, in a flexed position, while the procedure is in progress.
- Lumbar punctures should not be implemented when there is evidence of a raised intracranial pressure. It will lower the pressure at the base of the spinal cord while the brain still has fluid at high pressure. This variance in pressure can cause the brain to be pulled downwards into an area of restricted space. The brainstem will be compressed and life is threatened.
- Strict aseptic technique must be used for this procedure.
- Check the puncture site for leaking cerebrospinal fluid.
- A specimen of venous blood should be taken at the same time as the lumbar puncture for comparison.
- It is normally a requirement that the patient should lay flat in bed for 6–8 hours after this procedure, to prevent or reduce the potential for post-lumbar puncture headache.
- As a period of bedrest in the recumbent position is normally required following lumbar puncture, it is advisable that, if possible, the patient uses the toilet before the procedure.
- Specimens must be sent to the laboratory immediately.

CONTAINER

The specimen containers used in this unit are:

PURPOSE

To examine the cerebrospinal fluid for:
- Deviation from normal component and pressure values
- The presence of abnormal materials.

Cerebrospinal fluid circulates around the brain and spinal cord providing a shock-absorbing cushion against:
- The inflexible bone skull in which the brain is enclosed
- Injuries to the head.

It is contained between two layers of the meninges in the subarachnoid space.

This fluid barrier enclosing the brain and spinal cord maintains a stable environment in which the central nervous system can operate. Irregularities may occur in the blood and tissues but the effects on the brain are delayed by the protective barrier of cerebrospinal fluid.

NORMAL PHYSIOLOGY

Cerebrospinal fluid is formed at the site of each choroid plexus in the ventricles of the brain. A choroid plexus is a collection of blood vessels which are covered with cells that have the ability to constantly manufacture and secrete cerebrospinal fluid.

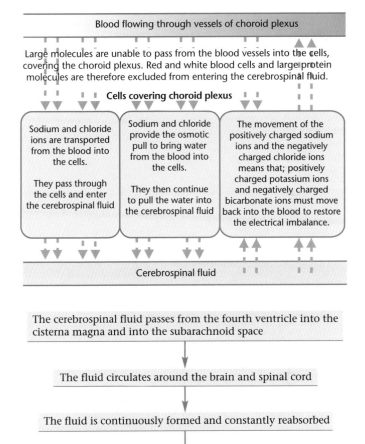

Blood flowing through vessels of choroid plexus

Large molecules are unable to pass from the blood vessels into the cells, covering the choroid plexus. Red and white blood cells and large protein molecules are therefore excluded from entering the cerebrospinal fluid.

Cells covering choroid plexus

Sodium and chloride ions are transported from the blood into the cells. They pass through the cells and enter the cerebrospinal fluid	Sodium and chloride provide the osmotic pull to bring water from the blood into the cells. They then continue to pull the water into the cerebrospinal fluid	The movement of the positively charged sodium ions and the negatively charged chloride ions means that; positively charged potassium ions and negatively charged bicarbonate ions must move back into the blood to restore the electrical imbalance.

Cerebrospinal fluid

The cerebrospinal fluid passes from the fourth ventricle into the cisterna magna and into the subarachnoid space

↓

The fluid circulates around the brain and spinal cord

↓

The fluid is continuously formed and constantly reabsorbed

↓

The subarachnoid space has projections that enter the venous sinuses: the arachnoid villi

↓

The arachnoid villi give the close proximity of cerebrospinal fluid and venous blood needed for the reabsorption of cerebrospinal fluid back into the blood

ALTERED VALUES

COLOUR

Clear, colourless
- Normal cerebrospinal fluid
- Viral meningitis
- Degenerative nerve disease, e.g. motor neurone disease

Cloudy, turbid
- Raised white blood cell content:
  - Presence of bacterial infection, e.g. bacterial meningitis
  - Intracranial tumour
- Burst intracranial abscess

Red
- Blood contamination from insertion of spinal needle
- Recent haemorrhage into subarachnoid space, e.g.
  - Ruptured cerebral aneurysm
  - Subarachnoid haemorrhage

Yellow
- Xanthochromia, bile pigments from haemolysis, evidence of a past haemorrhage into the subarachnoid space
- High protein content

PRESSURE

Lumbar puncture should be avoided when there is evidence of raised intracranial pressure.

Factors that influence the pressure of cerebrospinal fluid

The volume of circulating cerebrospinal fluid
- The arachnoid villi are unable to absorb the cerebrospinal fluid back into the venous system of the blood
  - Congenital condition causing hydrocephalus
  - Damage to arachnoid villi by neoplasm

The presence of additional substances in the circulating fluid
- Transport mechanisms of the absorbing cells blocked by abnormal components of the cerebrospinal fluid
- Increased matter circulating as part of the cerebrospinal fluid, e.g.
  - Increased cell count as a reaction to an inflammatory or infectious disorder

Obstruction to the flow of cerebrospinal fluid
- A tumour may block the flow of cerebrospinal fluid, raising the measured pressure
- When the tumour is in the spinal cord, cerebrospinal fluid pressure above the obstruction can be raised but the pressure below the obstruction may be lower than normal

Venous pressure
- If the blood pressure in the veins of the arachnoid villi is high, the water from the cerebrospinal fluid will not be able to use hydrostatic pressure to return to the blood. The volume of cerebrospinal fluid will not be reduced.

BLOOD CELLS

A minimal presence of lymphocytes are the only blood cells that are usually found in the cerebrospinal fluid.

Red blood cells and white blood cells

- Contamination of the cerebrospinal fluid with blood following insertion of the spinal needle during the lumbar puncture
- Haemorrhage into the subarachnoid space:
  - Subarachnoid haemorrhage
  - Ruptured cerebral aneurysm

White blood cells
An increased presence of white blood cells in the cerebrospinal fluid signifies an immune reaction to cerebral infection or inflammation.

Polymorphonucleocytes
- Bacterial meningitis
- Early viral meningitis
- Leptospiral meningitis

Lymphocytes
- Viral meningitis
- Tuberculous meningitis
- Viral encephalitis
- Carcinoma of the brain or meninges

Monocytes
- Aseptic meningitis
- Multiple sclerosis
- Neoplasms

NEUROLOGICAL CELLS

Neurological cells will be found in the cerebrospinal fluid following surgical or accidental trauma.

GLUCOSE

Glucose passes from the blood into the cerebrospinal fluid as it is formed by the choroid plexuses.

The normal value of glucose in the cerebrospinal fluid is 50%–66% of blood glucose.

A blood glucose measurement should be taken concurrently with the lumbar puncture to compare results.

Increased glucose levels

Disturbances of glucose diffusion into the cerebrospinal fluid:
- Hyperglycaemia
- Raised intracranial pressure

Decreased glucose levels

Bacteria use glucose for metabolic purposes.
The presence of bacteria will reduce glucose levels.
- Bacterial and tubercular meningitis
- Intracranial abscess

Altered values

PROTEIN

Measured cerebrospinal protein values will include albumin, globulin, fibrinogen and bacteria.

Most protein molecules are too large to pass from the blood into the cerebrospinal fluid at the choroid plexus.

Raised values of protein

Reaction to neurological infection or inflammation, e.g.
- Bacterial or viral meningitis
- Cerebral abscess
- Multiple sclerosis

Cerebral haemorrhage:
- Ruptured cerebral aneurysm
- Subarachnoid haemorrhage

CHLORIDE

There is a higher concentration of chloride in cerebrospinal fluid than in the blood.

UREA

Urea in cerebrospinal fluid remains at the same concentrations as blood urea.

Raised urea levels

Cerebrospinal fluid urea will rise above normal when blood urea rises.
- Uraemia

CALCIUM

Calcium levels in the cerebrospinal fluid are half the values of blood calcium.

Raised calcium values

Cerebrospinal fluid calcium values will rise as cerebrospinal fluid protein values rise as calcium is transported attached to protein molecules, e.g.
- Meningitis

ASSOCIATED INVESTIGATIONS

		Related pages
Temperature	Infection found in the cerebrospinal fluid will cause the temperature to rise.	4
Pulse	Raised intracranial pressure will reduce the rate of the pulse.	9
Blood pressure	Raised intracranial pressure will cause the blood pressure to rise.	17
Respirations	Increased pressure on the respiratory regulation centre in the brain from raised intracranial pressure or damage from 'coning' following the lumbar puncture will cause disruption or cessation of respiration.	129
Level of consciousness State of mind	Lumbar puncture is not an appropriate procedure when the patient shows evidence of raised intracranial pressure.	262
Equal size and reactivity of pupils Examination of the optic disc	When the fundus of the eye is examined with an ophthalmoscope, papilloedema or swelling of the optic disc will be seen when the intracranial pressure is raised.	253
Tone and power of muscular movement	Regular neurological examinations will give some indication of the severity and progress of the cerebral dysfunction.	
Infants – Occipital-frontal head circumference – Fontanelles	The unfused skull bones of a neonate or infant will be separated by the increased pressure of circulating cerebrospinal fluid beneath them. The head will enlarge. When the intracranial pressure is raised, the fontanelles on the skull of the neonate or infant will bulge and feel tense when touched.	
Assessment of the cranial nerves	Each of the 12 cranial nerves are specific to the normal function of identifiable parts of the body.	245
Skull X-ray Ultrasound brain scan Computerised tomography Magnetic resonance imaging Cerebral angiography	Imaging of the brain to identify defects or damage.	295 298
Posture	Meningism, Kernig's sign.	245
Cisternal puncture	Removal of cerebrospinal fluid from the cisterna magna. The needle is placed just below the occipital bone.	

CONSIDERATIONS FOR CARE

RAISED CEREBROSPINAL FLUID PRESSURE (HYDROCEPHALUS)

A rise in cerebrospinal fluid pressure within the chamber of the skull can cause distortion and compression of brain tissue. As pressure increases on areas of brain tissue, correct body function will be disrupted. Life support mechanisms may be at risk.

It is essential for a planned, multidisciplinary approach to care. Movement and intrusive procedures will increase cerebral irritation. A policy of minimal handling should operate.

The neurological health of the patient must be monitored by measuring and recording:
- Levels of orientation and consciousness
- Tone, power and symmetry of muscular movement
- Pupil size, bilateral equivalence and reactivity to light
- The vital signs:
  - Temperature – damage to the temperature regulation centre or presence of infection
  - Pulse – a decreasing pulse is an indication of increasing cerebrospinal fluid pressure
  - Blood pressure – a rising blood pressure is an indication of a rising cerebrospinal pressure
  - Respirations – damage to the respiratory centre will cause changes to respiratory patterns.

Headache can be a problem. Analgesia, if given, must be chosen carefully. It must not mask deterioration in the patient's condition or induce further drowsiness. Covered ice-packs laid on the head may ease the pain.

Visual disturbances, if they occur, will be a source of anxiety to the patient and family. Supportive care is essential to explain this and the other disturbing features of this condition.
Explanations that can be understood must be given to describe the steps being taken to alleviate the condition.

A raised cerebrospinal fluid pressure may also induce vomiting. It can be projectile and often without the warning of nausea. To keep the area fresh and to improve the patient's comfort the patient's skin must be kept clean; good, effective mouth care will be needed; and clothing, bedlinen and bedroom must be cleaned as necessary.

An accurate fluid intake and output chart will be required to record the vomiting, and assist in the assessment and monitoring of the patient's hydration and nutrition.

In infants, whose skull bones have not yet fused and in whom the skull is capable of expanding, regular measurements of the occipital-frontal head circumference will monitor increasing pressure.

If the hydrocephalus does not resolve, surgical procedures to relieve the pressure may be considered. Local policy of pre-operative preparations must then be followed.

NEUROLOGICAL EXAMINATION

PURPOSE

To assess the ability of the brain and nervous system to provide appropriate, co-ordinated body function.

PROCEDURE

Interviewing the patient

The interview is best conducted with a close friend or relative of the patient present. They can be supportive to the patient and staff by providing corroborative or additional information. Their presence is obviously essential when the patient is unable to provide a coherent explanation for themselves.

The purpose of the questions will be to establish:
- The normal pattern and structures of the patient's life
- Family, social and cultural background
- Known physical defects
- Any relevant factors in the medical history of the patient or his or her family
- The reason for the patient or his or her relatives to seek help.

Information taken from this conversation may contain:
- A foundation for the comparison of presenting features with a usual mode of behaviour
- Indicators that may explain the neurological changes, i.e. genetic disorders
- Factors that have to be taken into account when the neurological assessment is conducted, i.e. deafness rather than confused thinking as a possible cause of irrational answers.

Responses from the patient need to be considered in conjunction with:
- The patient's appearance and mannerisms
- The patient's grasp of place and time
- The rationality of the answers
- The patient's demeanour
- Short- and long-term memory
- Manner and tone of speech.

Physical examination

- Assessment of the patient's level of consciousness. Set criteria should be used to measure the level of consciousness against an agreed gauge, e.g. the Glasgow Coma Scale
- Stimulus needed to elicit a response
- Ability to obey requests or commands
- Appropriate eye opening and eye contact
- Posture, gait and co-ordination
- Recognition of objects, reading and writing
- Abnormal movements:
  - Muscle tremors or twitches
  - Decerebrate movement – one or both arms and legs extended rigidly
  - Decorticate movement – one or both arms bent across the chest, legs extended

- Muscle tone and power:
  - Spastic, flaccid or rigidity
  - Loss of power
  - Muscle atrophy
  - Neck stiffness
- Fine movements and precision location.

Romberg's test
The patient is asked to stand with his or her feet together and eyes open for 30 seconds then the patient is requested to close his or her eyes for 30 seconds.

Swaying occurs under normal circumstances but a positive test occurs when the patient needs to move their feet in order to regain balance.

Tests of sensory function
These will evaluate peripheral nerves and the sensory pathways of the spinal cord.

Assessment should test the patient's ability to recognise the presence of stimulus, discriminate between points of the body where the stimulus is placed and differentiate between a variety of sensations.

Areas of the body that show an exaggerated or reduced reaction, or absence of reaction, should be recorded.

The sensations tested should include:
- Touch – a light touch to the skin
- Deep pressure – pressure on a tendon
- Vibration – with the use of a tuning fork
- Temperature – distinguish between warmth and cold
- Pain – using both ends of a pin, distinguish between a sharp and blunt object
- Proprioception – a consciousness of the body position
- Two point discrimination – how far apart two identical points, simultaneously applied, need to be before discrimination between one point and two can take place.

Reflex responses
Two types:
- Superficial reflexes – a response to a sensitive area of skin
- Deep tendon reflexes – the tapping of a tendon will cause the tendon and its associated muscle to stretch. The reflex response to this sudden movement will stimulate the muscle to contract.

The responses should be graded, as exaggerated, normal, diminished or absent.

A full list of reflexes are found on pages 259–261.

Reflexes are very important to the neurological examination of neonates and infants.

Neurological signs
Kernig's sign – an indicator of meningeal irritation.
- The patient lies on his or her back
- The examiner puts his or her hands behind the patient's head and brings the head forward
- If the head resists the movement, or the patient's knees flex, the test result is positive.

Brudzinski's sign – an indicator of meningeal irritation.
- The patient lies on his or her back
- The examiner lifts one of the patient's legs forming a 90 degree angle with the hip and knee

- The knee is then straightened
- If the patient reports pain or resists the movement, the test result is positive.

Measurement of the occipital-frontal diameter of the skull
In neonates and infants, the unfixed skull bones will allow an increase in head diameter when an increased intracranial pressure exerts a force beneath them.

The adult skull diameter can be enlarged by disease, i.e. Paget's disease.

The shape of the neonatal skull
Signs of birth trauma should be identified:
- Abnormal skull shape caused by excessive moulding
- Caput – a swelling produced by prolonged pressure against the foetal head in the birth canal
- Cephalhaematoma – a swelling produced by a collection of blood under the periosteum of the skull bones, produced by prolonged pressure against the foetal head in the birth canal.

Fontanelles
The anterior and posterior spaces on the foetal skull between bone edges will close at about 18 months.

When raised intracranial pressure is apparent, the anterior fontanelle will become tense and bulging.

The vital signs
Temperature
A raised temperature may indicate:
- Infection
- Damage to the temperature-regulating centre.

A lowered temperature may indicate:
- Depression of the nervous system, through an overdose of drugs
- Hypothermia.

Pulse
A raised pulse may indicate:
- Haemorrhage
- A shocked state.

A lowered pulse may indicate:
- Raised intracranial pressure.

Blood pressure
A raised blood pressure may indicate raised intracranial pressure.
A lowered blood pressure may indicate a shocked state.

Respirations
A lowered state of consciousness may cause obstructed breathing.
Keeping a patent airway is vital.

Assessment of the 12 paired cranial nerves

I	The olfactory nerve	A sensory nerve. Gives a sense of smell.	■ Ensure that the patient can smell and identify test odours.
II	The optic nerve	A sensory nerve. Gives vision.	■ Visual acuity – object recognition or ability to read. ■ Visual fields – test of peripheral vision. ■ Colour recognition.
III	The occulomotor nerve	A motor nerve. Raises the eyelid. Constricts the pupil. Supplies some muscles that give the eye movement.	■ Test of ability to open the eye. ■ Test of pupillary reflexes to light. ■ Test for divergent eye movement.
IV	The trochlear nerve	A motor nerve. Supplies some muscles that give the eye movement.	■ Test for divergent eye movement.
V	The trigeminal nerve	A sensory nerve to touch. Ophthalmic branch Maxillary branch Mandibular branch	Test touch responses bilaterally to: ■ Cornea ■ Forehead, cheeks ■ Jaws.
		A motor nerve for mastication.	■ Test strength and positioning of jaw movement.
VI	The abducens nerve	A motor nerve. Supplies some muscles that give eye movement.	■ Test for divergent eye movement.
VII	The facial nerve	A sensory nerve to taste. A motor nerve for facial expression.	■ Test of taste identification. ■ Test strength of facial muscles against resistance.
VIII	The acoustic nerve	A sensory nerve. Cochlear branch Vestibular branch	Tests to assess: ■ Hearing ■ Balance and posture.
IX	Glossopharyngeal nerve	A sensory nerve for taste, and for touch to pharynx, soft palate and tonsils.	■ Identification of tastes. ■ The presence of the gag reflex.
		A motor nerve for swallowing, talking and salivation.	■ Assess movement of the soft palate.

X	The vagus nerve	A sensory nerve for larynx and posterior ear. A motor nerve for pharynx, larynx and upper oesophagus. Parasympathetic nerve supply to the heart and intestines.	Test for the presence of: ■ Gag reflex ■ Cough reflex ■ Ability to swallow. Assess sensation and movement of the soft palate. The quality of the voice.
XI	The spinal accessory nerve	A motor nerve. Turns the head and neck. Shrugs the shoulders. Moves the soft palate.	Test head, neck and shoulder movements against resistance.
XII	Hypoglossal nerve	A motor nerve. Controls the tongue.	Assess the tongue for movement and symmetry.

ASSOCIATED INVESTIGATIONS

		Related pages
White cell count	A differential count will show the presence of an inflammation or an infection.	**44**
Blood glucose	Neurological changes can be caused by abnormal blood glucose values.	**85**
Lumbar puncture	The tapping of the lumbar spine to collect a specimen of cerebrospinal fluid for laboratory analysis.	**238**
Cisternal puncture	Removal of cerebrospinal fluid from the cisterna magna. The needle is placed just below the occipital bone.	
Continuous intracranial pressure monitoring	A pressure-sensitive probe is placed in the intracranial cavity.	
Carotid Doppler ultrasonography	Uses ultrasound technique to assess the blood flow through the carotid arteries, to the brain.	
Skull X-ray	Taken from various angles, the X-ray can only show disease that has had an impact on the bone of the skull, i.e. fractures, bony erosions, tumours of the skull.	**295**
Electroencephalogram	The electrical tracings recording brain activity.	
Cerebral angiography	The imaging of the cerebral blood vessels on X-ray, after the injection of a contrast medium into the cerebral circulation. Distortion of the vessels can indicate tumours, aneurysms, stenosis, occlusions, abscesses and injuries.	**295**
Air encephalogram	The imaging of the fluid spaces around and within the brain – the ventricles and subarachnoid space. Obstruction to the flow of cerebrospinal fluid can be located. Brain size can also be measured.	
Brain scan	A picture of the brain will be developed according to the amount of radioactive dye taken up by the brain cells. Lesions within the brain will become obvious as abnormal brain tissue takes up more of the dye than normal tissue.	
Computerised tomography	This computerised analysis of radiographic imaging will show a wide variety of cerebral tissue abnormalities.	**296**
Single photon emission computed tomography	The radionucleotide used is able to pass through the blood–brain barrier. From this, a detailed picture of blood flow through the brain can be recorded.	
Magnetic resonance imaging	A process that presents a differentiated image of soft tissue in addition to the more compact tissues.	
Electromyography	Takes a recording of electrical impulses passing through skeletal muscles as a way of detecting peripheral nerve dysfunction.	

CONSIDERATIONS FOR CARE

Neurological damage or disease can threaten the patient's ability to maintain their own airway.
Correct positioning to prevent airway obstruction and constant monitoring of respiratory effort will be needed.

Monitoring of temperature, pulse, respiration and blood pressure will alert the nurse to other changes in the life-support mechanisms.

Monitoring neurological changes using the level of consciousness, orientation, pupil reactions and the ability to move and respond are also needed to look for signs of improvement or deterioration in neurological function.

Signs of a rising intracranial pressure may also include headache, stiff neck, vomiting, visual disturbances and convulsions.

When signs of raised intracranial pressure become obvious, action must be immediate. The fact that a positive sign has appeared means that brain tissue is being compressed and distorted. The tissue will become ischaemic and damaged.

When neurological debility changes the personality or elements of the mind that make up the unique person, it is extremely difficult and confusing for the patient and their family.
The patient's room should have memory-jogging photographs around it. Pictures of the patient taken before the neurological changes happened will remind the patient, family and staff of the real identity of the person before the change in behaviour. Their favourite music should be played and familiar voices must speak to the patient.

When reduced consciousness or confusion are part of the neurological problem, introducing a structure to the patient's day can begin the process of reorientation.

Communications with the patient must be clear and simple, and loud enough to hear. Although the patient may appear to be deeply unconscious, verbal warnings must be given prior to any care or contact.
When a response from the patient is requested or expected, allow adequate time for reply.

Hospitals can be insular places even for fully orientated patients. For neurologically damaged people the isolation can be a cause of disorientation. The day, date and time, weather and other news should all be part of the information given to the patient over the day.

The dignity of the patient may lie entirely in the hands of the carers. They must guard it at all times.

Skin care will become important. Reduced consciousness or the inability to move will put increased pressure on areas of skin. Regular movement will be needed to relieve that pressure. Pressure-reducing, weight-bearing mattresses and chair seat covers will be needed. Sheets on which they lie or sit must be free of creases.

The skin must be kept clean and dry. Barrier creams should be used if the skin is likely to become wet through incontinence. These should be applied gently, without rubbing.

Other benefits of movement:
- Keeping muscle tone and preventing muscle atrophy
- Stimulating the circulation of blood
- Helping to move and expel mucous secretions from the airways.

Considerations for care

When patients are unable to move for themselves, it is important that they are made comfortable in their new position, each limb is properly supported and that they are completely safe.

The diet must ensure that sufficient nutrients are available for body maintenance and repair.
The method of nutrition will depend on the patient's ability to swallow, and the presence of an adequate gag reflex.

Increased dietary fibre or bowel preparations must be given if needed to keep the regular bowel movement.

Rehabilitation is a major part of the process of recovery when cerebral tissue has been damaged.

All the caring agencies concerned with the patient and their family must become part of an agreed plan for the return to a maximum degree of normal life.

EXAMINATION OF THE PUPILS

NORMAL MEASUREMENT

The pupils of the eye must:
- Be equal in size
- React briskly to light
- Maintain identical diameters at all times.

PROCEDURE

Having a light shone into the eyes can be uncomfortable and distressing.

Children, especially, may react badly to the procedure. Game playing, and involvement of the child's parents as providers of support and comfort, may avoid or reduce the child's distress.

Reactions of the pupils to light may need to be tested throughout the night and can become very irritating to the sleeping patient. The procedure must be completed quickly and competently with the minimum of disturbance. The patient's reaction to the procedure will often give information on the level of arousal and awareness to record on the neurological chart.

PURPOSE

A raised intracranial pressure interferes with normal pupillary responses.

Increased pressure on the brain and nerve routes supplying the pupils will cause them to become unequal in size and fail to respond to light.

The pupils of the eye alter in size according to the amount of light entering the eye.
The pupil gets smaller as the amount of light increases – the pupillary light reflex. The pupil also constricts when focusing on a close object.

Both pupils must be of equal size when examined. They must constrict in unison as the light is passed over each eye, constricting to the same size, at the same rate.

Other assessments to be made:
- Consensual constriction – both pupils react uniformly and identically.
- Convergence constriction – pupils constrict and converge when focusing on an object held at nose level and brought slowly closer to the face.
- Correct open position of the eyelid – The eyelid is raised by the action of the oculomotor nerve, cranial nerve number III. When impulses are unable to travel along this nerve, the eyelid stays in the lowered position. This is termed ptosis.

NORMAL PHYSIOLOGY AND REASONS FOR ABNORMAL REACTIONS

Light enters the pupil of the eye.
Nerve cells of the retina respond to bright light.

Nerve impulses are sent along the optic nerve, cranial nerve number II.

The optic nerve joins the eye at the site of the optic disc or the blind spot on the retina. → Raised intracranial pressure will cause pressure on the optic nerve.
The pressure produces a swollen or choked optic disc, seen when the retina is examined using an ophthalmoscope.
This is papilloedema.

The nerve fibres from each eye meet and some fibres cross sides at the optic chiasma.
The nerve fibres separate once again into two branches.

The branches are sent to opposite sides of the brain.

The optic nerve ends at the occipital cortex of the brain.
A group of optic nerve fibres also end in the mid-brain.

It is from these mid-brain fibres that the oculomotor nerve, cranial nerve number III, is stimulated to send parasympathetic nerve impulses to the eye to constrict the pupil – miosis.

→ Unilateral dilated, fixed pupil
– The oculomotor nerve becomes compressed by abnormal shifts of brain tissue on the damaged side. Tissue moved by increasing intracranial pressure.
– The pressure on the nerve prevents it from sending impulses along its length. The pupil is unable to constrict.
– The fixed pupil appears on the same side as the area of brain damage.

Bilaterally dilated, fixed pupils
– Severe brain damage
– Brain death.

When insufficient light is entering the retina or pupil dilatation is needed for focus, nervous impulses stimulate the cervical ganglion of the paravertebral ganglionic chain. → Interruption of the sympathetic nerve pathways will cause the pupils to constrict and remain constricted – pinpoint pupils.

Sympathetic nerve impulses return to the eye and the pupil dilates – mydriasis.

ABNORMAL FEATURES

STRABISMUS – UNCOORDINATED EYE MOVEMENTS

Both pupils should follow identical paths of movement and direction.

Damage or disruption to nerve or muscle fibres to the eye will cause unsynchronised movement.

NYSTAGMUS – UNEVEN EYE MOVEMENT

Movements of the eyes should be smooth.

Damage or disruption to nerve or muscle fibres that control eye movements can cause a jerky eye motion.

SETTING SUN PUPILS

The downward direction of the iris of the eye and the band of visible white sclera above resemble a setting sun.

It is seen in infants with hydrocephalus.

OCULOCEPHALIC REFLEX – DOLL'S EYE REFLEX

- Normal reaction – as the head is turned, the pupils of the eye move in the opposite direction:
    - Head turned to left – eyes move to the right
    - Head turned to right – eyes move to the left
    - Nod head up and down – eyes move up and down in opposite direction.
- Abnormal reaction – as the head is turned, the pupils remain centred without the corresponding movement in either direction.

The absence of this reflex indicates severe brain or brainstem damage, even brain death.

VISUAL FIELD DEFECTS

Nerve fibres serve the retina to provide a complete picture of our surroundings.

The fibres originate as the optic nerve at the common point of the optic disc, seen on the retina.

As the optic nerve travels back to its point of contact with the brain, nerve fibres responsible for particular visual fields, i.e. upper fields and lower fields, leave the optic nerve for their own particular control area in the brain.

When these specific nerve fibres or their area of brain tissue is not functioning correctly, the visual field that they serve will be affected.

Abnormal features

ARGYLL ROBERTSON PUPIL

A small pupil that fails to constrict to light but will constrict on convergence.

It may be a sign of neurosyphilis.

CALORIC OR VESTIBULAR-OCULAR REFLEX

A test to establish a functioning brainstem or brain death.

Ice-cold water is trickled into the ear. If the brainstem is functioning the pupils of the eye will turn away from the affected ear.

CORNEAL REFLEX

The patient is asked to look to one side. The cornea on the opposite side of the eye is touched lightly with a soft material. This should produce a blink.

An infant should turn its head towards a light

YELLOW SCLERAE

Associated with jaundice. Discoloration by excessive amounts of bile pigments in the blood.

ARCUS SENILIS

An opaque ring around the cornea.

It appears with old age. Its presence in younger people can be an indication of hyperlipidaemia.

BITOT'S SPOTS

White triangular marks on the cornea.

A sign of vitamin A deficiency.

NORMAL MEASUREMENT

Reflex testing should be evaluated against an agreed response scale.

PROCEDURE

A stimulus is provided to elicit two types of reflex response:
- A deep tendon reflex – the tapping of a tendon to stimulate a muscle contraction.
  An examination of the spinal reflex arc.
- Superficial reflexes – an area of skin or mucous membrane is provoked to produce an expected response.
  An examination of spinal and cortical nerve pathways.

PURPOSE

To assess the effectiveness of the nerve pathways supplying the tested areas of the body.

Some reflexes are essential to the survival of the newborn. This protection continues into maturity, as reflexes give rapid defensive responses when the body experiences danger. Reflexive movements also help muscles to work co-operatively to maintain an upright stance.

The rapid response of the reflex reaction depends mainly on the direct action reflex arc that passes through the spinal cord.
The reflex stimulus also initiates activity along the nerve pathways ascending the spinal cord to the brain to invoke further appropriate reactive responses.

Reflexes test the transmission of nervous impulses in a very direct, measurable way.
An exaggerated, diminished or absent response can help to indicate the point where nerve pathways are reduced or severed.

Each tested reflex will be limited to one side of the body only. Bilaterally corresponding reflexes should be symmetrical in speed and degree of response.

The progress of a neurological disorder can be monitored by recording reflex responses throughout the course of the disease, on a set scale.

NORMAL PHYSIOLOGY

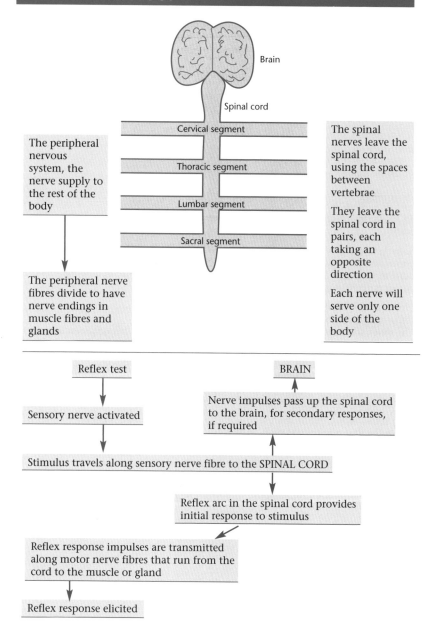

The peripheral nervous system, the nerve supply to the rest of the body

The peripheral nerve fibres divide to have nerve endings in muscle fibres and glands

Brain

Spinal cord

Cervical segment

Thoracic segment

Lumbar segment

Sacral segment

The spinal nerves leave the spinal cord, using the spaces between vertebrae

They leave the spinal cord in pairs, each taking an opposite direction

Each nerve will serve only one side of the body

Reflex test

Sensory nerve activated

BRAIN

Nerve impulses pass up the spinal cord to the brain, for secondary responses, if required

Stimulus travels along sensory nerve fibre to the SPINAL CORD

Reflex arc in the spinal cord provides initial response to stimulus

Reflex response impulses are transmitted along motor nerve fibres that run from the cord to the muscle or gland

Reflex response elicited

INFANT REFLEXES

In health, babies are born with their own set of reflexes. These reflexes will disappear as the cortical region of the brain develops and the baby gains neurological maturity.

Sucking reflex   When a nipple or teat is held to a baby's mouth, the baby responds by opening the mouth and sucking.

Rooting reflex   When a corner of the mouth or the cheek is touched, the baby will turn its head towards the touched side and open its mouth.

Tonic neck reflex   When lying down with head to one side, the baby will extend the arm on the side of the turned head and flex the knee on the opposite side.

Grasp reflex   When the palm of a baby's hand is touched, the fingers grasp the object.
The same response occurs when the soles of their feet are touched; the toes curl to grasp the object.

Babinski reflex   When the sole of the foot is stroked, the great toe pulls upwards and the toes fan outwards.

Walking reflex   When the baby is held upright with their feet touching a surface, the baby will lift one leg and move it as if to make a step.

Response to light   When a light is held at one side of a baby's head, it will turn its head towards that side.

An infant will also have the protective reflexes listed on the next page.

CHILD AND ADULT REFLEXES

The protective reflexes of:
- Swallowing
- Vomiting
- Cough
- Gagging
- Sneeze

Deep tendon reflexes

Biceps reflex	Tested at the inside bend of the elbow
Triceps reflex	Tested on the outside bend of the elbow
Brachioradialis reflex	Tested on the wrist
Patella reflex	Tested on the knee
Achilles tendon reflex	Tested at the back of the heel

Superficial reflexes

At the umbilicus
Stroking the skin across the abdomen at the umbilicus causes the umbilicus to move.

Cremasteric reflex
When the inner thigh of a male patient is stroked, the testicle on that side rises.

Plantar reflex
The lateral aspect of the sole of the foot is stroked.
- Normal reaction – the toes curl downwards
- Abnormal reaction – the great toe pulls upwards and the other toes flare outwards (Babinski's sign).

Gluteal reflex
Stroking the skin of the buttocks causes the underlying muscles to contract.

Withdrawal reflex
When the skin records the sensation of heat or pain, that point of the body is rapidly withdrawn from the source of harm.

Palmomental reflex
The skin on the palm of the hand near the thumb is stroked.
- Abnormal reaction – a wrinkling of the skin of the chin on the stroked side. May occur with Parkinson's disease.

Glabellar reflex
The bone just above the nose is tapped.
- Abnormal reaction – continuous blinking or the eyes remain shut.
May occur with Parkinson's disease.

Scapular reflex
Stroking the skin in the interscapular region will cause the scapulae to contract.

Child and adult reflexes

Eye reflexes

Reactive pupils
When light is shone into the eyes, the pupils constrict.

The pupils constrict when accommodating to close objects.

Oculocephalic reflex
■ Normal reaction – when the head is turned, the eyes move in the opposite direction.
As the head is nodded downwards, the eyes roll upwards.
As the head is nodded upwards, the eyes roll downwards.
■ Abnormal reaction – the eyes remain static and centred as the head is moved in any direction.

Corneal reflex
The eye blinks when the cornea is touched.

Caloric oculo-vestibular reflex
When ice water is trickled into the ear, the eyes are seen to move in a direction away from the tested ear.

Excretory reflexes

Defaecation
■ It is the reflex action brought about by faeces entering the rectum that produces defaecation.
■ The filling of the rectum causes stretching of the rectal walls.
■ This stimulates a reflex wave of peristalsis to travel from the descending and sigmoid colon.
■ The anal sphincter relaxes and the faeces are expelled.
■ Nerve transmissions from the brain delay the defaecation response until it is socially acceptable for the defaecation reflex to operate.

Micturition
■ It is the reflex action brought about by urine entering the bladder that produces a micturition.
■ The filling of the bladder causes stretching of the bladder wall. This produces a reflex that causes the bladder wall to contract. As the bladder becomes more full, the reflex and responding muscle contractions cause the bladder to be in a state of strong contraction.
■ Nerve transmissions from the brain delay the bladder emptying until socially acceptable conditions are available to pass urine.

Diving reflex

A response to the head being submerged in water.
■ Bradycardia
■ Vasoconstriction
■ Reduced oxygen requirements to tissues.

This reflex increases the survival time if at risk of drowning.

LEVEL OF CONSCIOUSNESS

NORMAL MEASUREMENT

To have an awareness of oneself, and to have appropriate, alert responsiveness to surroundings and stimulus.

PROCEDURE

When there is a deterioration from full consciousness, a frequent estimation of the level of consciousness should be made and recorded.

These measurements must be taken using an approved neurological assessment standard.

The measurements usually taken to quantify the degree of unconsciousness are based on the amount of stimulus needed, and the quality of the responses to elicit an opening eye, a verbal response and a motor response from the patient.

A baby or a young child will need a grading tool appropriate to their maturity and normal responses.

PURPOSE

To grade the degree of unconsciousness, and monitor changes of awareness and responsiveness.

The reticular activating system found in the brainstem is a channel for all sensory nerve impulses entering the brain from the spinal cord. It channels some of these messages up to the cerebral cortex for a response to be initiated and sent back down the nerve pathways for appropriate action to be taken.

It is the reticular activating system that keeps the body in a state of consciousness.

The state of consciousness declines when:
- The reticular activating system is unable to function correctly
- The cerebral cortex has failed and is unable to produce responses to sensory input.

The care of a patient with reduced consciousness should be driven by the need to:
- Maintain a patent airway
- Protect the body from further damage
- Treat the reason for the onset of coma, if appropriate.

CAUSES OF UNCONSCIOUSNESS

REASONS FOR REDUCED CONSCIOUSNESS

Neurological	Non-neurological
Cerebral oedema	Drug overdose
Herniation	Poisoning
Cerebral vascular disease	Diabetes mellitus
– Haemorrhage	Hypothermia
– Embolism	Anoxia
– Thrombosis	Myxoedema
Infection	Liver failure
– Encephalitis	Renal failure
– Meningitis	Metabolic disease of the newborn
Trauma	Anaesthesia
Space occupying lesions	
Seizures, fits	

When the cause of unconsciousness is unknown the patient must be examined for explanatory clues:

■ A history taken from a friend or relative
■ The smell of the breath, e.g.
  – Acetone breath with ketosis
  – Alcohol
■ Signs of bruising or trauma
■ Needle marks on the skin
■ Rashes, e.g.
  – Petechia with meningitis
■ Leakage of cerebrospinal fluid from the nose or ear
■ Blood tests, e.g.
  – Blood glucose value.

WEIGHT

REFERENCE RANGE

Adult: A body mass index of 20.1–25.0.

The body mass index is calculated from: $\dfrac{\text{Weight (kg)}}{\text{Height (m)}^2}$.

Child: Children's growth should be within percentile lines on an appropriate weight and height growth chart.

Neonate: The expected weight will vary according to the gestational age. An average weight for a term, 40-week, baby is 3163 g ± 595 g.

PROCEDURE

Standing or sitting scales for adults and children.
Sitting or laying scales for babies and infants.

Accurate weight can only be measured when all clothes are removed.
When a child or infant is weighed, play or distraction may be needed to keep them still and happy during the procedure.

When serial weighing is needed the measurement must be taken:
- At the same time each day, preferably early morning before the patient has eaten
- Wearing the same clothes, if any are worn
- On the same weighing scales.

PURPOSE

To check that the patient's weight is within accepted limits, set by age, height and frame.

The control of the deposition of fat is affected by many physiological factors. Surplus intakes of fats, carbohydrates and proteins may be stored in the body as fat. The energy sources from foods eaten should equal energy expended for a stable body weight.

The normal intake of food is controlled by the feeding centre of the hypo-thalamus. It gives the feeling of hunger and the feeling of satiation when enough has been eaten.

Appetite for food will override these feelings. Loss of appetite will prevent food intake even when the body needs to eat. The body will depend on its fat deposits for energy and they will become depleted. A large appetite will take in more food than the body needs and the fat deposits will grow.

Weight is part of a combination of tests for nutritional assessment:
- Height is taken to calculate the body mass index
- Skinfold thickness measured with callipers
- The mid-arm circumference.

The pattern and distribution of the fat deposits should be noted.

NORMAL PHYSIOLOGY

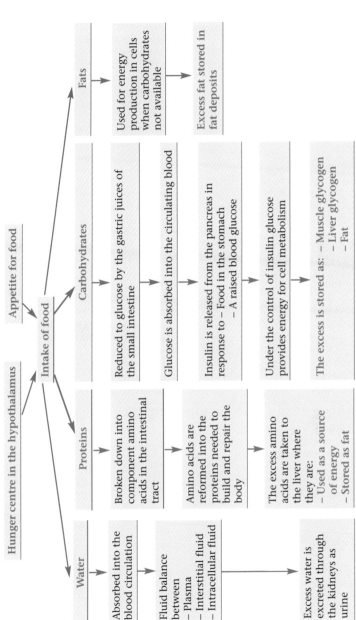

Hunger centre in the hypothalamus | **Appetite for food**

Intake of food

Water
- Absorbed into the blood circulation
- Fluid balance between
  - Plasma
  - Interstitial fluid
  - Intracellular fluid
- Excess water is excreted through the kidneys as urine

Proteins
- Broken down into component amino acids in the intestinal tract
- Amino acids are reformed into the proteins needed to build and repair the body
- The excess amino acids are taken to the liver where they are:
  - Used as a source of energy
  - Stored as fat

Carbohydrates
- Reduced to glucose by the gastric juices of the small intestine
- Glucose is absorbed into the circulating blood
- Insulin is released from the pancreas in response to – Food in the stomach – A raised blood glucose
- Under the control of insulin glucose provides energy for cell metabolism
- The excess is stored as: – Muscle glycogen – Liver glycogen – Fat

Fats
- Used for energy production in cells when carbohydrates not available
- Excess fat stored in fat deposits

Fat stores are broken down for use when the body can no longer use carbohydrates for the production of energy to fuel cell metabolism.

ABNORMAL WEIGHT GAIN AND LOSS

WEIGHT GAIN	WEIGHT LOSS
Fluid retention	**Dehydration**
Excessive food intake	Inadequate food intake
	Physical causes
Destruction or damage to the hypothalamic feeding centre	Destruction or damage to the hypothalamic feeding centre
	– Loss of appetite through illness or drug therapy
Increased number of fat cells acquired in childhood	– Nausea
	– Food intolerance and allergies
	– Dieting
Enlargement of fat cells as an adult	
Psychogenic causes	Psychogenic causes
– Comfort eating	– Anorexia nervosa
	– Depression, anxiety
Environmental	Environmental
– Overeating as an acquired habit	– Starvation
	– Poverty
	– Immobility
	The use of fats for cell metabolism
	The inability to metabolise glucose
	– Diabetes mellitus
Decreased energy expenditure to food intake	Increased energy expenditure to food intake
Metabolic causes	Hyperthyroidism
– Hypothyroidism	
– Hypersecretion of the adrenal glands, Cushing's syndrome	
Effects of drugs, including:	
– Corticosteroids	

ASSOCIATED INVESTIGATIONS

		Related pages
Haemoglobin	A test that reflects the quality and the quantity of food intake.	38
Total protein Serum albumin	Will decrease when protein intake is insufficient.	72 75
Blood urea	Urea is the waste product of protein metabolism. Blood urea will rise with a high protein diet and fall with a low protein diet.	121
Urine tests ■ Glucose ■ Ketones	Test for diabetes mellitus, a cause of weight loss. Present in the urine when fat is used for energy production.	193 197
Skinfold thickness Body circumference	Measured with callipers. Needs to be measured at the same points of the body each time.	
The skin	Signs of dehydration, poor condition, sores and signs of poor wound healing.	269
The mouth and mucous membranes	The hygiene of the mouth and the ability to eat. Sores around the mouth.	
Fluid intake and output	Prevents dehydration. Records the patient's willingness to take drinks.	
Routine weighing	To keep a record of weight gain or weight loss.	

CONSIDERATIONS FOR CARE

The size of the body has a major influence on self-image. It can affect self-esteem and confidence, two factors that can affect the volume of food taken each day. Comfort eating or dieting in excess lead to abnormal body weights.

The choice and amount of food, and the times that it is taken, usually follow long held habits.

Breaking a regular practice is difficult. Modification of existing practices will have a more lasting impact for change.

The patient's co-operation will be needed when dietary habits have to be changed. The need to appreciate the reason for the change in diet is essential or it will become a hopeless exercise. Education and counselling regarding the benefits of keeping to the diet can help.

The diet must be food that the patient can afford, shop for locally and prepare easily. The patient must find the food appetising and acceptable in the patient's culture. The texture of the food suggested must be within the patient's physical ability to eat it. Dental treatment may be necessary.

A dietitian will be an essential source of help and advice.

When the diet is part of a patient's treatment, the food offered must be attractively presented and in the correct proportions. Checks must be made on the portions eaten and the portions left on the plate. The amount of food eaten at each meal should be recorded.

Refusing to eat can signify deep psychological problems. Individual and family therapy will need to be part of the strategy when trying to normalise eating habits.

Special attention to diet must be paid to people who rely on others to feed them. The food must be presented with utensils that allow the patient the maximum degree of independence to feed themselves. If feeding is necessary, the patient must not feel hurried; neither should they feel a loss of dignity.

The food must not be left to go cold while dinners are handed to more able eaters. Good conversation to accompany the food always helps this social event.

Carers must be vigilant when food is withheld from patients, i.e. pre-operatively and post-operatively. Food provides the essential ingredients for healing. The patient's nutritional status must be constantly monitored and other methods of keeping the patient nourished must be found.

EXAMINATION OF THE SKIN

NORMAL MEASUREMENT

Normal findings will be defined by the patient's personal characteristics of age, race and state of health.

PROCEDURE

Examination of the skin requires:
- A good light
- A warm environment for comfort
- When sensitive areas of the body are exposed, modesty blankets are used to preserve the patient's dignity.

PURPOSE

The skin is examined for marks and signs that imply systemic or local disorders.

The formal examination of the skin is constantly augmented by the observations made by staff during their contact with the patient. Carers can not avoid close contacts with the patient's skin when implementing treatments and procedures. Careful observation of the skin will give valuable clues to the present and potential well-being of the patient.

The functions of the skin are numerous. It also serves to give each person an identity.

It places people into racial and age groups. It can be a sign of social class, employment and be a reflection of the patient's way of life.

Changes occurring in the skin chart progress through life. This may become a challenge to the patient's self-image. Abrupt changes occurring through accident or disease will be especially hard to cope with.

Every individual carries unique skin characteristics, i.e. birthmarks, moles, skin tone.

An ageing skin will have less elasticity and vascularity than a child's skin. These changes mean that adjustments have to be made when considering what would be acceptable normal or abnormal findings.

Examination of the hair, the nails and mucous membranes should also be part of the assessment.

NORMAL PHYSIOLOGY

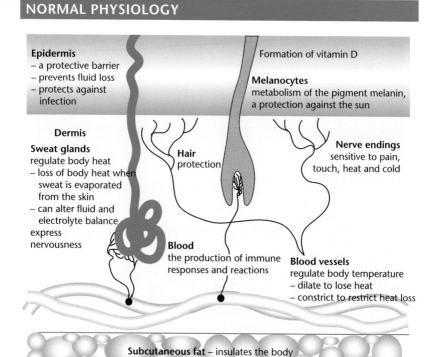

Epidermis
– a protective barrier
– prevents fluid loss
– protects against infection

Formation of vitamin D

Melanocytes
metabolism of the pigment melanin, a protection against the sun

Dermis

Sweat glands
regulate body heat
– loss of body heat when sweat is evaporated from the skin
– can alter fluid and electrolyte balance
express nervousness

Hair
protection

Nerve endings
sensitive to pain, touch, heat and cold

Blood
the production of immune responses and reactions

Blood vessels
regulate body temperature
– dilate to lose heat
– constrict to restrict heat loss

Subcutaneous fat – insulates the body
– stores fat until it is needed as a metabolic fuel

Skin – normal function

OTHER FEATURES FOR ASSESSMENT

Odour

The presence of body odour is one of the first assessments that can be made when close contact is made with the patient. Causes are:
- Nervous sweating due to stress of examination
- Poor hygiene
- Incontinence.

Sensitive or tender areas of skin

Numbness or paraesthesia

Pruritis, itching skin

Generalised:
- Uraemia
- Liver failure.

Localised:
- Urticaria.

Bruises and scars

Oedema

Hair

- Condition and cleanliness
- Has the normal male or female distribution and patterning.

Rashes

There are many types and patterns of skin lesions that may be described as a rash.

Points of significance when lesions are apparent:
- Other signs of disease
- Recent food and drug intake
- Recent stress
- Areas of the body affected
- Size, shape and features of the lesions.

Lesions, ulcers, moles

The skin can present the examiner with a multitude of marks, injuries and lesions.

The examiner must determine:
- The origin of the abnormality
- The nature of the advice and treatment already given
- The nature of any changes seen in the lesion
- The symmetry of distribution on the skin.

The butterfly rash of systemic lupus erythematosus:
- An erythematosus rash spreading across the bridge of the nose and outwards across both cheeks.

Spider naevii with chronic liver failure:
- A branching superficial arteriole.

ASSESSMENT OF COLOUR

Normal skin colour will depend on:
- The amount of skin pigment produced by melanocytes
- The amount of blood circulating in the skin.

Pallor

A pale or white skin.
- Blood vessels in the dermis are constricted, reducing the flow of blood:
  - Cold – constricting the blood vessels of the skin will reduce heat loss.
  - Stress or shock – causes the sympathetic nervous system (adrenaline) to constrict the blood vessels of the skin. Blood becomes redirected to organs that may need extra supplies of oxygen during the time of crisis.
- Anaemia – a reduction of the haemoglobin content of the blood.
- Obstruction to the blood flow supplying the skin:
  - Obstructive disease of the main or peripheral blood vessels supplying the skin.
- **Circumoral pallor** – A ring of pale skin around the mouth.

Cyanosis

Blueness of the skin.
An increased amount of unoxygenated haemoglobin is circulating in the blood.
- A failure of the respiratory system to supply the blood with oxygen, or a failure of the heart to circulate oxygenated blood. This will cause **central cyanosis**, as the lips and tongue become blue as well as the skin.
- Slow-moving blood through the skin of the periphery will be depleted of its oxygen by the surrounding tissues. This produces **peripheral cyanosis**:
  - Constricted blood vessels from cold or shock
  - Inadequate pumping of the blood through the peripheral circulation
  - Obstructive disease of the peripheral circulation.

Mottled skin

The skin is not a uniform colour; the skin has a red or bluish patterning.
- There is a reduction in the blood filling the capillary blood vessels of the skin
- A reduced blood haemoglobin.

Flushed or red skin

- The blood vessels in the dermis are dilated to lose heat through the skin.
- Raised body temperature through infection, climate or exercise.
- Inflammation causes capillary blood vessels in the dermis to become engorged with blood. This causes localised areas of redness or **erythema**.
  - Infection
  - Sunburn
  - Inflammatory conditions.
- Polycythaemia vera – an excess of red blood cells gives a bluish tinge to the redness.

Jaundice	A yellow skin colour. An increased amount of bilirubin in the blood causes the skin and the sclera of the eyes to become yellow in colour. ■ An increased breakdown of red blood cells – haemolytic jaundice. ■ There is a normal pathway taken by bile. Manufactured in the liver, it moves through the bile ducts to the gall bladder for storage. When needed, it moves down the common bile duct into the small intestine. Liver disease or obstruction of the bile ducts can cause bile to pass into the blood circulation – cholestatic jaundice. ■ Congenital hyperbilirubinaemias – non-haemolytic jaundice.
Bronze	■ Tanned by the sun ■ Addison's disease ■ Pernicious anaemia, the combination of haemolytic jaundice and the resulting anaemia.
Yellow-brown	■ Chronic renal failure, retention of pigments normally passed out in the urine.
Lack or loss of skin pigment	■ Albinism – a lack of melanin. Can be localised patches or apply to the whole body. ■ Vitiligo – areas of the skin lose their melanocytes, leaving white patches. Cause unknown.
Haemorrhage of the skin	■ Fresh or old bruising.

ASSESSMENT BY TOUCH

Temperature of the skin	Variables that affect the temperature of the skin: ■ The degree of capillary dilation in the dermis ■ The amount of blood filling the capillaries. Skin temperature should be considered in association with: ■ Skin colour ■ Amount of moisture felt on the skin ■ Signs of local or generalised infection or inflammation ■ Asymmetrical temperature differences in the limbs.
Warm or hot skin	Dilated capillary blood vessels in the dermis increasing heat loss from the body. ■ Infection ■ Exercise ■ Climate. Increased volume of blood in the capillaries of the dermis in response to a localised area of inflammation.
Warm wet skin	Areas of the body vary in their ability to sweat. Assessment should note whether the sweating is generalised or confined to certain areas of the body. ■ Sweating as a mechanism to lose body heat ■ Sweating as a nervous response – sympathetic nervous reaction to stress.
Cold skin	Constricted capillary blood vessels in the dermis: ■ Reducing heat loss from the body – hypothermia ■ Redirection of blood to the vital organs – shock. Occlusion of the arterial blood supply to a limb will reduce the temperature of the limb.
Cold wet skin (clammy)	■ Blood vessels of the dermis constrict to increase blood flow to the vital organs. ■ Sweating is increased by the sympathetic nervous system response to stress: – Shock.
Dry skin	■ Cold environment preventing the need to sweat ■ Dehydration ■ Poor nutrition ■ Hypothyroidism.
Capillary refill	A test of the ability of peripheral capillary vessels to fill with circulating blood. When pressure is applied to an area of skin or a nail bed, blood flow to that area is obstructed and the site becomes white or blanched. The pressure is released, and the time is recorded for the skin to return to normal colour. The normal response occurs within 3 seconds.
Skin elasticity	Age reduces the elasticity of skin, as the collagen fibres in the dermis gradually become less effective.

Skin turgor, the amount of water in the tissues of the skin, also affects the elastic recoil of the skin.

When a fold of skin is pinched, the time taken for it to return to normal position will demonstrate its degree of elasticity. Age allowances need to be made against the expected recoil time.

Increased recoil time

■ The elderly
■ Decreased skin turgor, a reduction in the water content of skin tissues:
– Dehydration.

Oedema or swelling

The skin becomes stretched and shiny over a swollen area of skin.

The skin may indent when pressure from a finger is applied to it – pitting oedema.

Note must be taken of:
■ The areas of the body that are oedematous
■ Whether the oedematous areas are symmetrical
■ Colour of the skin over the oedematous areas
■ Other signs of disease shown by the patient.

Oedema is caused by excessive amounts of water collecting in or below the skin tissue.

It has localised and general causes. The sites and distribution of the oedema will usually indicate the underlying cause.

Causes are:
■ Poor blood circulating capability, local to a body area of the central circulation
■ An inflammatory reaction, a localised response
■ Poor lymphatic drainage from an area of the body
■ High levels of sodium in the interstitial tissues.

Nails

Nails should be inspected for:
■ Ridging – transverse ridges indicate that previous disease had temporarily stopped the nail from growing
■ Pitting – abnormal indentations
■ Inflammation in the nail fold or around the cuticle, paranychia
■ Absent nails
■ Haemorrhage under the nails – from trauma or vascular disease
■ The degree of hardness – signs of brittleness, softness, split nails
■ Shape of the nail – spoon shaped: koilongchia associated with anaemia
– clubbing of nails: an expanded end of finger tip and an excessively curved nail, associated with chronic hypoxia of peripheral tissue.

ASSOCIATED INVESTIGATIONS

		Related pages
Temperature	A flushed skin is commonly associated with a raised temperature. Hypothermia will cause a pale or mottled skin.	**4**
Haemoglobin Red blood cell count	Anaemia causes a pallid complexion. A raised red cell count or polycythaemia will cause a florid complexion.	**38** **34**
White cell count	To determine the presence of infectious disease.	**44**
Erythrocyte sedimentation rate	Will be raised with inflammatory skin disease.	**43**
Urine test for glucose	Increased urine glucose may cause pruritis around the urethral meatus.	**193**
Swabs for culture and sensitivity	To test the exudate from a lesion for the presence of infective organisms.	**294**
Blood clotting tests	Bruising may be significant when blood clotting mechanisms are defective.	**63** **66**
Skin scrapings	For cytology, for identification of parasites and fungal infections.	
Sensitivity tests	The skin is used to test the body's sensitivity to potential allergens.	
Skin biopsy	To identify the basis of a skin lesion.	

CONSIDERATIONS FOR CARE

Skin is an important reflection of personality and identity.

When disease or accident alters the skin or appearance, sensitive support must augment the physical tasks of caring to help the patient adapt to the new condition.

Changes in the skin also give important information that alert the carer to the patient's needs.
- The skin will reflect a poor nutritional state.
  This will affect wound healing and recovery time.
  Preventative measures will be needed to avoid further skin damage, especially when the patient is immobile and pressure areas are at risk.
- The skin will reflect allergies.
  The warning given by the appearance of a skin rash will alert patients and carers to the sensitivity. Avoiding the allergen will avoid the more serious effect of anaphylactic shock.
- The skin will reflect the need for better hygiene.
  This will be a personal matter for most people and tact will be needed when trying to help patients improve their hygiene routine.
  The responsibility for patient cleanliness often lies with the carers and they must be diligent when caring for the skin, especially when incontinence or excessive diaphoresis are part of the condition.
  Feeling clean often helps with the patient's feeling of well-being.
  Body odour or knowledge that a wash is needed will cause unnecessary embarrassment to the patient.
  Help with bathing and skin care following use of the toilet must be performed ensuring that the patient's dignity is retained as a priority.

Tissue reacts to injury by showing the inflammatory response.

Initiators of the inflammatory response can be chemical, i.e. drugs or allergens, or trauma.

The purpose of the response is to:
- Localise the injury
- Counteract the causative agent
- Tissue repair.

The visible signs of inflammation following injury to tissue are:
- Redness
- Pain
- Heat
- Swelling.

Other signs of an inflammatory response are:
- Wheals or red swollen marks on the skin – the triple response
- Itching or urticaria
- Angioneurotic oedema, a life-threatening condition causing swelling of the skin, mucous membranes or the larynx
- Anaphylactic shock.

THE TRIPLE RESPONSE MECHANISM

The local response to a tissue injury.

A line of pressure drawn across the skin releases histamine from the tissues.

1st response

There is localised vasodilation and a **red** mark appears on the skin. Vasodilation produces increased **heat** loss from the wound.

2nd response

A bright red border surrounds the red skin mark.

3rd response

The released histamine causes the walls of the dilated capillaries to have increased permeability. Fluid therefore leaks into the injured tissues. The red line on the skin becomes **swollen** and it becomes a wheal.

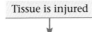

Tissue is injured

Histamine is released by mast cells at the site of the injury
Vasoconstriction of the capillary blood vessels occurs at site of reaction
The area of injury becomes red and hot

Histamine:
– Dilates the capillary blood vessels
– Causes bronchoconstriction during anaphylactic shock
– Increases the permeability of the dilated capillary blood vessels

Dilation of the capillary blood vessels at the site of the reaction:
– Increased blood flow – area becomes red and hot

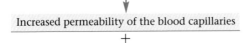

Increased permeability of the blood capillaries
+
Increased hydrostatic pressure within the capillaries

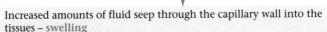

Increased amounts of fluid seep through the capillary wall into the tissues – swelling

The swelling stimulates the nerve endings – pain

The fluid contains:
– Red blood cells
– White blood cells
– Platelets
– Antibodies
– Fibrinogen.

The blood clotting factors seal off the area of injury preventing further tissue movement.

The white blood cells:
– Stimulate the immune response
– Phagocytose the invading organisms
– Clear away debris at the site of injury.

The immune response may cause a rise in body temperature.

LIFE-THREATENING INFLAMMATORY RESPONSES

Angioneurotic oedema

Swelling of the skin and mucous membranes that may lead to laryngeal obstruction.

Anaphylactic shock

A reaction to a protein, usually a drug or a food, to which the body has become sensitive. The foreign protein stimulates the IgE antibodies. The increased number of IgE antibodies attach themselves to the mast cells and cause large amounts of histamine and other substances to be released. The blood pressure falls and anaphylactic shock may follow.

ASSOCIATED INVESTIGATIONS

COMPLEMENT FIXATION TESTS

Complement is a group of circulating proteins that work with antibodies to destroy harmful antigens, i.e. bacteria.

Complement:
- Ruptures the cell membranes of the bacteria
- Causes the surrounding mast cells to release more histamine increasing the inflammatory reaction
- Has the ability to attract phagocytic white cells to the area of injury
- Causes organisms to become more susceptible to the action of phagocytes, speeding the destruction of the antigen and the removal of debris.

Complement fixation tests are used to detect the presence and the proportions of an antibody–antigen reaction. An identified antibody or antigen is added to a sample of the patient's serum. The serum is incubated. If an antibody–antigen reaction is active in the patient's serum, the complement present in the sample will be used up. If no reaction occurs, complement will remain unused in the sample. Therefore, when red blood cells coated with the same antibody or antigen are added to the serum:
- The red cells will break down if complement is still present
- The red cells will remain intact if the complement has been exhausted.

MONOCLONAL ANTIBODY ASSAYS

These tests are used for identifying and typing cells, including antigens.

In the presence of an antigen, B-lymphocytes generate numerous identical antibodies.

The laboratory generates specific antibody–antigen reactions and harvests the antibody produced. Cells carrying the antibody are kept in conditions where they can proliferate.

They can then be used as a basis for tests of cell identification.

IMMUNOFLUORESCENCE

A technique to identify many of the substances present and generated when an immune response is taking place.

A dye is added to the specimen, which becomes attached to antibodies present. The antibodies are fluorescent when viewed under an ultraviolet microscope.

RADIOIMMUNOASSAY

This test measures the amount of antigen in a specimen of serum.

A specific quantity of a marked antigen and amounts of unmarked antigen are added to the serum. Both are in competition for binding sites on the antibodies present in the serum. A graph is drawn measuring the amount of binding by the labelled antigen before the addition of each quantity of unmarked antigen.

The graph will show how much of the patient's antigen was already in the sample.

C-REACTIVE PROTEIN

REFERENCE RANGE

C-reactive protein is not normally present in blood.

PROCEDURE

Venepuncture.

CONTAINER

The specimen container used in this unit is:

PURPOSE

To determine whether C-reactive protein has appeared in the blood.

C-reactive protein is a globin produced by the liver when antibodies are formed in response to inflammation, bacterial infection or tissue trauma. It appears within a few hours of the onset of tissue inflammation and damage. It does not provide specific causal information, but it will indicate the presence of one or more of these generalised conditions. Sequential measurements will indicate the phasing of recovery.

Intrauterine contraceptive devices and oral contraceptives may give a false positive result and anti-inflammatory drugs – i.e. steroids, salicylates and non-steroidal anti-inflammatory drugs – may initiate a false negative result.

ASSOCIATED INVESTIGATIONS

		Related pages
Erythrocyte sedimentation rate	Another measure of the presence of inflammation or infection.	**43**
Differential white cell count	A rise in a specified type of white blood cell may indicate the cause of the raised C-reactive protein.	**44**
Temperature	The presence of an infection will cause a rise in temperature.	**4**
Swabs and cultures	Specimens that detect the source and type of infection. The infective organisms' sensitivity to antibiotics will also be tested.	**292**
Assessment of symptoms		

Oedema is the abnormal collection of fluid in the body tissues.

The skin is examined for signs of swelling.

The skin over the swollen area may be:
- Pale, tense and shiny
- Red with inflammation.

The swelling can be general or local to a particular area of the body.

Swelling is part of the inflammatory response to injury and allergy. Areas of local swelling should be examined for signs of internal or external injury.

Gravity may affect the site of the oedema. The fluid collects at the lowest points of the body, i.e. the ankles when sitting or standing, the sacrum when lying or sitting in bed. This is dependent oedema.

Pressure with the thumb, above a bone, on an area of swollen skin may produce an indentation that is visible after the thumb is removed. This is pitting oedema. The amount of fluid accumulated in the tissues will determine the depth of the pitting.

Pitting oedema is normally associated with cardiac dysfunction.

Oedema in the abdominal cavity is termed ascites.

If a large amount of oedema is in the abdominal cavity, 'a fluid wave' will be felt on one side of the abdomen, when the examiner taps the opposite side. Regular, recorded abdominal girth measurements will detect an increase or reduction in the amount of collected fluid. Guide marks placed on the skin to position the tape measure correctly will ensure that measurements are taken around the same body diameter each time.

Oedema in the lungs, pulmonary oedema, will reduce the oxygen and carbon dioxide transfer capability of the lungs.

Cerebral oedema, a response to intracranial damage, will cause the brain to swell. The brain tissue has a limited area for expansion inside the hard bony skull. If the swollen brain tissue becomes compressed inside the vault of the skull, injury to brain tissue will be increased and life is threatened.

NORMAL FLUID TISSUE BALANCE

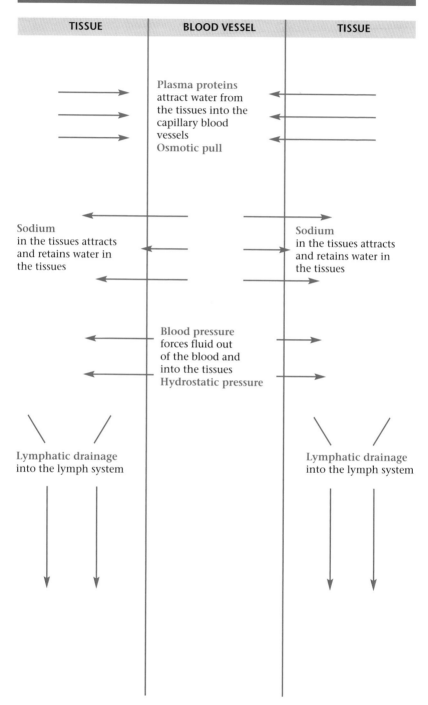

THE DEVELOPMENT OF OEDEMA

TISSUE	BLOOD CAPILLARY	TISSUE

Forces move fluid out of the capillary into the tissues

The forces that initiate fluid shift into the tissues are stronger than the forces that shift fluid back to the capillary

This results in tissue oedema or the filling of a body cavity with fluid

Lack of plasma proteins

Insufficient osmotic pull to bring the fluid back from the tissues

Raised contents of sodium in the tissues attract and retain too much water

Raised contents of sodium in the tissues attract and retain too much water

High capillary blood pressure

High pressures force increased amounts of fluid out of the blood vessel

Raised hydrostatic pressure

Walls of the capillary blood vessels alter to allow more fluid to pass through into the tissues

Blocked lymphatic tissue drainage

Blocked lymphatic tissue drainage

REASONS FOR OEDEMA

Lack of plasma proteins
– Malnutrition
– Loss of protein through the kidneys

High capillary blood pressure
– Inflammation
– Obstruction to venous flow away from the capillary
– Raised circulatory volume
– Prolonged standing or sitting

Capillary walls altered to allow more fluid to pass out of the blood vessel and into the tissues
– Anaphylactic shock
– Angioneurotic oedema
– Inflammation

Raised values of sodium in the tissues
– Cardiac failure
– Renal disease

Blocked lymphatic tissue drainage
– Surgery
– Infection
– Tumours
– Trauma

ASSOCIATED INVESTIGATIONS

		Related pages
Fluid balance chart	To record the fluid intake and the fluid output. This will give some indication of the amount of fluid retained by the body.	
Daily weighing	Large variations in the daily weight will suggest fluid retention or fluid loss.	264
Blood pressure	A rise in blood pressure may be linked with fluid retention and oedema. This especially applies in pregnancy. A measure of the cardiac output from a failing heart.	17
Electrocardiography Tests of cardiac function	To investigate heart disease as the basis of dependent oedema and pulmonary oedema.	24
Tests of renal function	To investigate renal disease as the basis of generalised oedema.	
Liver function tests	To investigate liver disease as the basis of ascites and generalised oedema.	
Lung function tests	To investigate the cause of pulmonary oedema.	
Blood protein value	Circulating protein attracts water from the tissues back into the blood. A lowered blood protein value would reduce the amount of fluid returning to the blood from the tissues.	72
Blood sodium value	Sodium attracts water. A rise in the value of sodium in the tissues will cause fluid to be retained. The tissues will become oedematous.	97

CONSIDERATIONS FOR CARE

Tissues carrying excessive volumes of fluid will become weakened. The fluid diminishes the supply of oxygen and nutrients reaching the cells. The stretched skin is easily damaged and will not have the ability to heal quickly.

These factors make pressure area care very important.

Unrelieved pressure or friction on oedematous skin will produce a sore area that will not resolve easily.

Oedema occurs or is made worse when the blood circulation is slow moving with poor venous return. Movement will activate the muscle pumps causing blood to circulate through the tissues more quickly. Walking, active and passive exercises must be encouraged.

Elastic support stockings will help prevent dependent oedema of the legs and feet.

Elevating the legs will also reduce oedematous legs, ankles and feet.

Tight bands must never be used around sites of oedema or a site of potential swelling. If the swelling increases, a complete circle of tape around a limb, finger or toe will act as a tourniquet, preventing the blood from flowing beyond the tape.

A programme of daily weighing will monitor the oedema. Fluid gained or lost will cause fluctuations in weight.

An accurate fluid intake and output chart will indicate fluid retention.

Diuretic therapy may be needed. If the extra fluid loss gives the patient a sense of urgency when they need to pass urine, easy access to a toilet will be necessary. There should be no delay when a bedpan or a commode is requested.

If the oedema is caused by sodium retention, a low sodium diet may be ordered.

A dietitian will give the necessary advice.

HUMAN IMMUNODEFICIENCY VIRUS

NORMAL MEASUREMENT

Enzyme-linked immunosorbent assay (ELISA) – no positive antibodies found.

Western blot test – no antibodies seen.

PROCEDURE

Venepuncture.

Before testing, discussion with the patient should highlight the benefits and disadvantages of having the test and knowing its result. Informed consent must be given prior to testing.

Protective gloves must be worn when taking the specimen of blood.

CONTAINER

The specimen container used in this unit is:

PURPOSE

To test for antibodies formed against the human immunodeficiency virus (HIV).

The ELISA test and the Western blot test are not totally reliable.

False-positive and false-negative results may occur.

Antibodies first start appearing in the blood 3 to 6 months after acquiring the infection.

Blood tests taken at this time may test negative. Another test 6 months after acquiring the infection will be necessary. This test may also be negative, despite the patient having the virus.

The HIV virus attacks the T4 lymphocytes. Having entered the blood circulation, the virus enters the lymphocyte and incorporates its genetic structure into the chromosomes of the white blood cell.

The virus can then remain dormant for many years.

When the T4 lymphocytes are stimulated and the cells use their chromosomes to divide and reproduce the cell, the virus will also be replicated.

The newly formed particles of HIV destroy the cell and attach themselves to other T4 lymphocytes and the sequence is repeated.

The destruction of the T4 lymphocytes weakens the immune system until the patient has very little protection against infection and malignant disease.

HIV infection becomes AIDS (acquired immune deficiency syndrome) when the immune system is unable to prevent the patient developing opportunistic infections or neoplastic conditions.

THE REPLICATION OF THE VIRUS

The virus enters the blood circulation.

HIV becomes attached to molecules on the surface of T4 lymphocytes.

The virus passes into the cell and enters the cell nucleus.

The nucleus of the cell contains genetic material.
This allows the cell to multiply and make identical copies of itself.
Replication is controlled by the double helix of DNA.
The DNA sequence of molecules is found on the cell's chromosomes.

Normally, when a cell divides, the DNA prescribes the molecular patterns that form.
HIV is a retrovirus, which incorporates into the genetic material of the cell.
HIV becomes the pattern for DNA to copy.
DNA alters its sequences of molecules to become identical to the sequence presented by the virus.

The virus becomes part of the genetic coding of the cell.
The virus is able to replicate itself using the lymphocyte's own DNA.
The cell begins to manufacture more HIV genetic material as cell particles.
The particles collect in the cells, making a path through to the surface of the cell.

The HIV granules burst the cell wall, killing the lymphocyte and dispersing more HIV genetic material into the blood circulation.

The cycle begins again as the particles attach themselves to more T4 lymphocytes.
More genetically coded particles are produced and more T4 lymphocytes are destroyed.

The immune system becomes unable to protect the body against harmful organisms.

CONSIDERATIONS FOR CARE

The consequences of testing for HIV need to be considered before a test is taken.

The benefits that a test can give are:
- The relief of anxiety when the test shows no infection
- If the test is positive, the patient will be aware that they are a source of infection to other people and make changes to prevent the spread of the disease
- The patient can receive appropriate anti-retroviral therapies.

The disadvantages of testing:
- The confirmation of HIV can confer sickness on an otherwise healthy person
- The positive test confirms the presence of a disease with a high mortality rate, a source of stress that is hard to come to terms with
- If patients are asked to confirm that a test had taken place, they may be put at financial and social disadvantage
- Attitudes of friends, family and colleagues may change towards the patient, if they knew that a test for HIV was needed. A positive result would risk greater impact on these relationships.

When it is known that the patient is HIV positive, they must be encouraged to take care of their health.

They must be aware of the resources that are available to them if worrying symptoms appear.

If the test is positive, the patient must understand how the virus is transmitted. They must be asked to use this knowledge to avoid infecting others.

SPECIMENS FOR CULTURE AND SENSITIVITY

PROCEDURES

Swabs and specimens for culture and antibiotic sensitivity.
- The specimen must not be contaminated:
  - Handle the specimen container on the outside only
  - Use aseptic techniques to collect the specimen
  - The specimen should not contain other substances, e.g. food particles.
- Wear gloves to handle the specimen container
- Recent and current antibiotic therapy should be reported on the laboratory slip
- Swabs should be taken from wet areas, collecting discharge and debris
- Swabs need to be in a transport medium for travel to a laboratory.

CONTAINER

The specimen containers used in this unit are:

PURPOSE

To identify organisms and specify the antibiotic that will destroy the infecting bacteria.

Gram's staining

Laboratory slides are smeared with material from the specimen taken.

The specimen is fixed to the slide. Colour dyes are put on to the slide and the bacteria take up their colour. The slides are then viewed under the microscope.

The bacteria are typed according to the stain they take:
- Gram-positive organisms take the purple stain of gentian violet
- Gram-negative organisms take the red stain of eosin.

Bacteria are also typed according to their shape when seen under the microscope:
- Rods or bacilli
- Cocci or round.

Acid-fast stain

A bacteria is described as acid fast when it stains with carbolfuchsin, after being washed with acid–alcohol solution.

Bacteria are also grouped into aerobic and anaerobic. An aerobic organism needs oxygen to live. Oxygen is detrimental to anaerobic bacteria.

Cultures

Culture mediums allow the organisms to feed and multiply under ideal conditions.

From this growth, firm identification of the invasive organism can be made.

Sensitivity

Once the infecting organism has been isolated, it is exposed to various antibiotics.

The bacteria may show:
- Resistance to an antibiotic that will not check its growth
- Moderate susceptibility to the antibiotic, which will slow its growth
- Sensitivity to the antibiotic that will destroy the bacteria.

The effective antibiotic can then be recommended as a treatment.

ASSOCIATED INVESTIGATIONS

		Related pages
Temperature	The presence of infection commonly causes a rise in temperature.	**4**
Pulse	The presence of infection may cause a rise in the pulse rate.	**9**
White blood cell count	The differential white cell count reflects the type of organism causing the infection.	**44**
An assessment of the infected area	To note areas of inflammation, discharges, presence of pus, smell, reporting of pain.	
Other symptoms of internal infections	Diarrhoea, vomiting, pain, lethargy.	
Complement fixation tests	Complement is a group of circulating proteins that helps the antibodies destroy antigens, i.e. bacteria.	**280**

CONSIDERATIONS FOR CARE

Specimens can be difficult to collect. The patient needs to understand the investigation and co-operate with its collection. A mid-stream urine collection is sometimes impossible.

Infection is a wide-ranging topic, and the specific care will be adapted to the type and site of the infection. The degree of generalised debility felt by the patient will alter the care requirements.

The infection may be a source of pain for the patient. Regular, effective analgesia should be offered.

Antipyretics should be offered when the infection causes a rise in temperature.

This is important when caring for a child under five, when a high temperature brings the risk of febrile convulsion.

The reduction of temperature and the relief of pain will make eating, drinking and movement more comfortable. If it is appropriate that the patient can maintain these activities, it will help prevent further complications caused by stasis, poor nourishment and dehydration.

The patient must be kept hydrated. Adequate nourishment will be essential to maintain the protein requirements of the immune system and for wound healing.

Practices that prevent cross-infection must be enforced.

Aseptic technique must be used when procedures are carried out on an infected site.

Contaminated material from the procedure must be disposed of safely and according to the local policy and practices.

Contaminated linen should be put in the appropriate coloured linen bag and labelled before disposal.

Local policy will list the infections that need complete isolation. Barrier nursing will then be practised. Isolation will not help to ease the patient's distress. Having to ring the call bell for every attention can become a source of stress.

The patient will need as much carer contact time as a patient in the open ward.

Antibiotic therapy is important. The course must be given in the right dose, at the right time each day until the end of the prescribed course.

X-RAYS

X-rays are used for screening and diagnostic purposes. They identify abnormal structures and incorrect positioning of organs.

X-rays are aimed at the part of the body that needs investigation. As the X-ray is taken, the radiation passes through the width of the body to form a picture on a film placed at the opposite side of the body.

As the X-rays pass through the body, the rays are interrupted by the internal structures encountered in their pathway. The X-rays that do reach the film turn the film black. The picture that forms is a negative image of the internal tissues.

The penetration of the tissues by X-ray depends on the density of the structures.
- Air and space allow the uninterrupted passage of X-rays. Air-filled cavities, i.e. lungs and flatus, look black on the X-ray picture.
- Organs and fat become a darker grey dependent on the ability of the X-rays to penetrate the tissue mass of the organ and reach the film.
- Water is a poor conductor of X-rays. Structures with a high water content look light on X-ray.
- Bones are impenetrable to X-rays. They will appear white on the X-ray picture.
- Dyes used to highlight particular tissues form an impenetrable barrier to X-rays. The contrasting white picture they make against the black film allows features to be seen that would not normally be visible.

X-rays are not without risk. They should be used with discretion. The procedure can be hazardous for patients and staff.

Protective screens and clothing must be worn by staff in close proximity to X-rays.

A radiation monitoring badge will be needed for staff who are in frequent contact with X-rays to monitor their exposure time. A pregnant woman should not be exposed to X-rays either as a patient or as a member of staff. If the slightest risk of pregnancy exists, conceived within the current menstrual cycle, it is important to avoid exposure to X-rays.

Some X-rays, especially those using contrast mediums, need the patient to be properly prepared.

The instructions from the radiography department must be complied with to avoid a poor image being produced and the patient having to return for a repeated procedure, and additional exposure to X-rays.

The carer attending a patient while an X-ray is being performed needs to be supportive and informative, to ease them through the procedure and obtain a good image.

When mobilisation or communication with the patient is difficult, the radiographer will appreciate the knowledge of the patient brought by the carer.

COMPUTERISED TOMOGRAPHY

Computerised tomography uses X-rays to make three-dimensional pictures of cross-sections of the body.

An X-ray machine revolves in an arc around the body of the patient. The pictures received reflect the varying density of the tissues met by the X-ray as they travel between the skin and the X-ray detector.

The images received are interpreted by a computer. It translates the X-ray information into pictures showing cross-sectional views of the body.

From these representations, tumours and other lesions, tissue damage, haemorrhage and tissue atrophy can be recognised.

Contrast mediums can be used to improve the quality of the pictures. An allergic reaction to the dye is possible.

Computerised tomography is a long procedure and the patient is required to lie completely still while it is producing the images. The patient must be safe and secure.

Sedation may be needed to relax the patient and help him or her to remain motionless.

Computerised tomography should not be used on a pregnant woman.

Preparation of the patient prior to the test will depend on instructions sent from the radiography department.

Discussions with the patient will be needed to explain the purpose of the test. Description of the test equipment and process can relieve some anxieties.

All metal objects and jewellery will need to be removed prior to the test.

Information specific to this department:

INVESTIGATIONS USING RADIOACTIVE MATERIALS

A radionuclide or a radioisotope is given to the patient. It is absorbed by the target organ. The radioactive material given will have an affinity with the organ to be tested and will be taken into its tissues.

The radioactive substance will act as a marker as it becomes part of the activity of the target organ.

A scanner is passed across the organ and a computer analyses the readings of radioactivity emanating from the scanned tissues. When high levels of radioactivity are recorded in one area it is described as a 'hot spot'. A low level of radioactivity is a 'cold spot'.

From this analysis, the size and outline of the structure can be assessed. The position of tumours, cysts and areas of non-functioning tissue are outlined.

Discussion with the patient needs to take place before the test. The patient has to know the time that the test will take, the preparations that need to be made and a description of the routine that will be followed.

The patient's own anxieties and queries must be addressed.

The radioactive substances will be excreted in the urine. To safeguard patients and staff, local guidelines and procedures must be followed when using the toilet, or disposing of a bedpan or commode subsequent to the investigation.

Information specific to this department:

ULTRASOUND TESTS

Ultrasound tests produce an image from ultrasound waves deflected from structures inside the body.

An electrical transducer is moved across the skin. The impulses from the transducer are changed into ultrasound waves as they travel through the internal organs.

When the ultrasound wave hits an internal structure it rebounds back to the skin.

The wave is altered back to electrical impulses by the transducer. A computer takes the incoming impulses and forms a picture. The imaging can be very rapid allowing motion from a beating heart or a foetus to be viewed.

Pretest preparations are usually employed to prepare the site for better penetration of the ultrasound waves, to obtain a better view of the target organs.

Discussions with the patient will need to include directions to prepare properly for the test and a description of the test procedure. Anxieties about the test will also need to be addressed.

Information specific to this department:

ENDOSCOPY

Endoscopes have been developed to give direct access to the hollow structures of the body.

Each endoscope is designed to enter a specified cavity. Once in place, the operator has a direct view of the structure. From this biopsies can be taken, and cautery and other local treatments can be given.

A camera can be attached and images produced. Endoscopic ultrasonography allows the examination of the full thickness of the lumen walls, through a transducer attached to the endoscope.

This identifies the presence of tumours and other abnormalities.

Endoscopy is an uncomfortable procedure if it is performed when the patient is fully conscious. Analgesia, sedation and local anaesthetics will help the patient to cope with the procedure.

Some endoscopies are performed under general anaesthetic, i.e. laparoscopy.

Preparation of the patient will need to follow the guidelines set by the local testing department.

The patient will need to be told of the test procedure and how they can co-operate with the endoscope operator to help the procedure along.

The patient will need to feel supported by the staff as the thought of these tests can be daunting and stressful.

After the test is completed, the patient must be certain that the endoscopy has not caused bleeding, either by perforating an organ or through taking biopsies.

Analgesia should be given for pain or discomfort felt as a result of the endoscopy.

When a local anaesthetic has been given to abolish the gag reflex, prior to endoscopic examination, food and fluids must be withheld until the reflex returns.

Information specific to this department:

HELPFUL INTERNET WEB SITES

For information on changes in available technology for assessment and nationally agreed reference ranges of normal values.

Department of Health, UK	www.doh.org.uk
Healthcare Commission	www.healthcarecommission.org.uk
Healthcare Development Agency	www.hda.nhs.uk
Medicines and Healthcare Products Regulatory Agency	www.mhra.gov.uk
National Health Service	www.nhs.uk
National Institute of Clinical Excellence	www.nice.org.uk
World Health Organization	www.who.int

HAEMATOLOGY

Erythrocyte sedimentation rate	<20 mm in 1 hour	The amount of sediment from blood cells that occurs in a tube of blood in a given period of time.
Haemoglobin	Male: 14–17.7 g/dl Female: 12.2–15.2 g/dl	The amount of haemoglobin contained in the red blood cells in a given quantity of blood.
Mean corpuscular haemoglobin concentration	32–35 g/dl	The average weight of haemoglobin in each blood cell.
Mean corpuscular haemoglobin	27–33 pg	The weight of the red blood cell.
Mean corpuscular volume	80–96 fl	The size of the red blood cells.
Packed cell volume (PCV) Haematocrit (HCT)	Male: 0.42–0.53 l/l Female: 0.32–0.45 l/l	The quantity of red blood cells expressed as a percentage of the total volume of blood.
Platelet count given	$150–400 \times 10^9$/l	The number of platelets in a volume of blood $\times 10^9$/l.
Red cell mass	Male: 25–35 ml/kg Female: 20–30 ml/kg	
Reticulocyte count	0.2–2.0% of RBCs	An immature red blood cell.
Serum B_{12} Serum folate Red cell folate	160–925 ng/l 4–18 µg/l 160–640 µg/l	Materials that are essential in the manufacture of red blood cells.
Serum ferritin	5.8–120 nmol/l	The amount of iron in depot for haemoglobin production.
Serum iron	13–32 µmol/l (70–175 µg/dl)	The iron bound to the protein transferrin, for transport in the plasma.
Total iron binding capacity	(45–72 µmol/l)	The total iron binding capacity of the blood: transferrin and other iron binding transport molecules.

White cell count	$4–11 \times 10^9/l$	The number of white cells, of all types, in a given quantity of blood.
Differential white cell count		Quantifies each type of white blood cell within a given amount of blood.
– Lymphocytes	$1.5–4.0 \times 10^9/l$	
– Neutrophils	$3.5–7.5 \times 10^9/l$	
– Monocytes	$0.2–0.8 \times 10^9/l$	
– Eosinophils	$0.04–0.4 \times 10^9/l$	
– Basophils	$<0.01–0.1 \times 10^9/l$	
Total blood volume	60–80 ml/kg	
Total plasma volume	40–50 ml/kg	

COAGULATION TESTS

Bleeding time	3–10 min	The time taken for bleeding to stop when the skin is pricked.
Activated partial thromboplastin time	30–50 s	Stimulates and assesses the capability of the blood clotting mechanism.
Prothrombin time	16–18 s	Time taken for blood to start clotting.
International normalised ratio (INR)	1	

BIOCHEMISTRY

Acid phosphatase	1–5 u/l	
Alanine aminotransferase	5–30 u/l	An enzyme that leaks into the blood from damaged liver cells.
Albumin	34–48 g/l	A plasma protein, made in the liver.
Alkaline phosphatase	25–115 u/l	Obstruction to the flow of bile causes the level of this enzyme to rise.
Alpha-1 antitrypsin	2–4 g/l	Decreased values may be associated with liver disease or emphysema.

Alpha-fetoprotein	<10 ku/l	Manufactured by the foetal liver. It is found in quantity in adults, liver disease and some neoplastic diseases.
Amylase	<220 u/l	An enzyme produced by the pancreas.
Angiotensin-converting enzyme	204–358 u/l	Angiotensin I is converted to angiotensin II by this enzyme.
Aspartate aminotransferase	10–40 u/l	Also called serum glutamic oxaloacetic transaminase (SGOT). Values of this enzyme rise when damage occurs to cardiac tissue, red blood cells, kidney, liver and lungs. The values rise according to the amount of damage.
Bicarbonate	22–30 mmol/l	Bicarbonate will change to maintain normal blood pH.
Bilirubin	<17 μmol/l	The breakdown product of red blood cells.
Caeruloplasmin	0.20–0.45 g/l	A globulin produced by the liver.
Calcium	2.20–2.67 mmol/l	Calcium is very mobile, moving between bone, plasma and tissues.
Carcino embryonic antigen		An antigen found during foetal life. Will re-appear when tissue healing is taking place or as a marker of the presence of a malignant tumour.
Chloride	100–106 mmol/l	A negative ion that provides electrical balance to positive sodium ions in the extracellular fluid.

Cholesterol	3.5–6.5 mmol/l	Cholesterol is synthesised by the liver and is taken in the diet.
HDL cholesterol	Male: 0.9–1.4 mmol/l Female: 1.2–1.7 mmol/l	High density lipoprotein.
Cholinesterase	2.25–7.0 u/l	Cholinesterase is an enzyme that breaks down acetylcholine. Acetylcholine links nerve endings to muscle fibres, generating muscle contraction.
Copper	12–25 μmol/l	Stored in the liver. Used in the manufacture of caeruloplasmin.
C-reactive protein	<10 mg/l	A protein probably made in the liver that appears in response to inflammation.
Creatinine	60–120 μmol/l	A product of anaerobic muscle metabolism.
Creatine kinase, cardiac	Female: 24–170 u/l Male: 24–194 u/l	An enzyme released when cardiac muscle is damaged by an infarction.
C_3	0.55–1.20 g/l	Part of the complement activation process leading to destruction of an invading organism.
C_4	0.20–0.50 g/l	Part of the complement activation process that leads to the destruction of an invading organism.
Ferritin	5.8–120 nmol/l	Absorbed iron is stored as ferritin.
Gamma glutamyl transpeptidase	Male: 11–50 u/l Female: 7–32 u/l	Raised values may be a sign of liver disease. Alcohol also raises the value above normal.

Glucose	4.5–5.6 mmol/l	Carbohydrates and sugars are digested for absorption into the blood as glucose.
Glucose-6-phosphate dehydrogenase screen		An enzyme of the red blood cell, essential for its normal life span.
Glycosylated haemoglobin	3.8–6.4%	Glucose molecules become attached to the haemoglobin molecule.
Hydroxybutyric dehydrogenase	40–150 u/l	An enzyme released from cardiac tissues following myocardial infarction.
Immunoglobulins – IgA – IgG – IgM	0.8–4 g/l 7.0–18.0 g/l 0.4–2.5 g/l	Elements of the body defence system.
Iron	13–32 μmol/l	Amount of iron absorbed into the circulation.
Lactate dehydrogenase	240–525 u/l	An enzyme released from cardiac tissues following myocardial infarction.
Lead	<1.2 μmol/l	
Lipids	4.0–10.0 g/l	The products of fat metabolism.
Lipoproteins – VLDL	0.128–0.645 mmol/l	Very low density lipoproteins
– LDL	1.55–4.4 mmol/l	Low density lipoproteins
– HDL	Male: 0.9–1.4 mmol/l Female: 1.2–1.7 mmol/l	High density lipoproteins
Magnesium	0.7–1.1 mmol/l	An electrolyte that pacifies nerve endings.
Non-esterified fatty acids	Male: 0.19–0.78 mmol/l Female: 0.06–0.9 mmol/l	
Osmolality	280–296 mosmol/kg	The osmotic pull of the solutes within a solution.
Phosphate	0.8–1.5 mmol/l	Phosphate and calcium ions share the same control mechanisms.

Phospholipid	2.9–5.2 mmol/l	
Potassium	3.5–5.0 mmol/l	A mainly intracellular electrolyte.
Sodium	135–146 mmol/l	A mainly extracellular electrolyte.
Total iron binding capacity	42–80 μmol/l	Measures the amount of transferrin available for the absorption and transport of iron.
Total protein	62–80 g/l	The total protein content of the blood.
Triglycerides	Male: 0.70–2.1 mmol/l Female: 0.50–1.70 mmol/l	Products of fat digestion.
Urate	180–420 μmol/l	The salt of uric acid.
Urea	2.5–6.7 mmol/l	The final product of protein metabolism. Excreted through the kidney.
Vitamin A	0.5–2.01 μmol/l	
Vitamin D 25-hydroxy 1,25-dihydroxy	37–200 nmol/l 60–108 pmol/l	
Zinc	7–18 μmol/l	Thought to be important in protein metabolism.

BLOOD GASES

Arterial P_{CO_2}	4.8–6.1 kPa 36–46 mmHg	The partial pressure of carbon dioxide in arterial blood.
Arterial P_{O_2}	10–13.3 kPa 75–100 mmHg	The partial pressure of oxygen in arterial blood.
Arterial $[H^+]$	35–45 nmol/l	Hydrogen ion concentration in arterial blood.
Arterial pH	7.35–7.45	

HORMONE LEVELS

Male
– Testosterone 10–35 nmol/l
– Luteinising hormone 1–10 ul/l
– Follicle-stimulating 1–7 ul/l
  hormone

– Sperm count
  – Volume 0.1–11 ml
  – Density 1.5–375 × 10^6 ml
  – Motility 5–95%

Female

– Testosterone 0.5–3.0 nmol/l

– Luteinising hormone Follicular 2.5–21 u/l
 Mid-cycle 25–70 u/l
 Luteal 1–10 u/l
 Post-menopausal >50 u/l

– Follicle stimulating Follicular 1–10 ul
  hormone Mid-cycle 6–25 u/l
 Luteal 0.3–21 u/l
 Post-menopausal >25 u/l

– Oestradiol Follicular <110 pmol/l
 Mid-cycle 500–1100 pmol/l
 Luteal 300–750 pmol/l
 Post-menopausal <150 pmol/l

– Progesterone Follicular <12 nmol/l
 Mid-cycle 0
 Luteal >30 nmol/l
 Post-menopausal <3 nmol/l

Total serum thyroxine (T4) 60–160 nmol/l

Total serum 1.2–3.1 nmol/l
tri-iodothyronine (T3)

Free serum thyroxine (T4) 13–30 pmol/l

Thyroid-stimulating 0.5–5.0 μl/l
hormone

	0900	2400 (asleep)
ACTH	10–80 ng/l	<10 ng/l
Cortisol	150–700 nmol/l	<150 nmol/l

Abramsky, L. and Chapple, J. (2003) Prenatal Diagnosis: The human side. Nelson Thornes, Cheltenham.

Beare, P., Rahr, V. and Ronshausen, C. (1985) Nursing Implications of Diagnostic Tests, 2nd edition. J.B. Lippincott Company, Philadelphia.

British Medical Association and the Royal Pharmaceutical Society of Great Britain (1995) British National Formulary. Number 29 (March). The Pharmaceutical Press.

Carrieri-Kohlmann, V., Lindsey, A.M. and West, C.M. (1993) Pathophysiological Phenomena in Nursing, 2nd edition. W.B. Saunders, London.

Chernecky, C., Kretch, R. and Berger, B. (1993) Laboratory Tests and Diagnostic Procedures. W.B. Saunders, London.

Colbert, D. (1993) Fundamentals of Clinical Physiology. Prentice Hall International (UK) Ltd, Hemel Hempstead.

Crawford, D. and Hickson, W. (2000) An Introduction to Neonatal Nursing Care. Nelson Thornes, Cheltenham.

Davison, A.M. (1988) Nephrology. Mainstream Medicine Series. Heinemann Medical Books, London.

Fishbach, F. (1992) A Manual of Laboratory and Diagnostic Tests, 4th edition. J.B. Lippincott Company, Pennsylvania.

Guyton, A. and Hall, J. (2001) Textbook of Medical Physiology, 10th edition. W.B. Saunders, Philadelphia.

Halliday, H., McClure, G. and Reid, M. (1989) Handbook of Neonatal Intensive Care, 3rd edition. Baillière Tindall, London.

Haslett, C., Chivers, E., Boon, N. and Colledge, N. (eds.) (2002) Davidson's Principles and Practice of Medicine, 19th edition. Churchill Livingstone, Edinburgh.

Higgins, C. (2000) Understanding Laboratory Investigations: A text for nurses and healthcare professionals. Blackwell Science, Oxford.

Hinchliff, S., Montague, S. and Watson, R. (1999) Physiology for Nursing Practice, 2nd edition. Baillière Tindall, London.

Kenner, C. and Wright Lott, J. (2003) Comprehensive Neonatal Nursing: A physiologic perspective, 3rd edition. Elsevier, Oxford.

Kumar, P. and Clark, M. (2002) Clinical Medicine, 5th edition. Baillière Tindall, London.

Levine, D.Z. (1991) Care of the Renal Patient, 2nd edition. W.B. Saunders, London.

Malasanos, L., Barkauskas V. and Stoltenberg-Allen, H. (1990) Health Assessment, 4th edition. The C.V. Mosby Company, St Louis, Missouri.

McGee, S. (2001) Evidence Based Physical Diagnosis. Saunders, Philadelphia.

McGhee, M.A. (1993) Guide to Laboratory Investigations, 2nd edition. Radcliffe Medical Press, Oxford.

Newell, R.G. (ed.) (1990) Clinical Urinalysis: The principles and practice of urine testing in the hospital and community. Ames Division Miles Limited, Buckinghamshire.

Provan, D. and Krentz, A. (2002) Oxford Handbook of Clinical and Laboratory Investigation. Oxford University Press, Oxford.

Skinner, S. (1996) Understanding Clinical Investigations, 1st edition. Baillière Tindall, London.

Vaughn, G. (1999) Understanding and Evaluating Common Laboratory Tests. Prentice Hall International (UK) Ltd, London.

Walsh, M. (2002) Watson's Clinical Nursing and Related Sciences, 6th edition. Baillière Tindall, London.

Weller, B. and Barlow, S. (1991) Paediatric Nursing, 7th edition. Nurses Aid Series. Baillière Tindall, London.

Weller, B. and Wells, R. (1990) Baillière Tindall Nurses' Dictionary, 21st edition. Baillière Tindall, London.

Wilson, D. (1999) Nurses' Guide to Understanding Laboratory and Diagnostic Tests. Lippincott, Philadelphia.